"Anyone can cheer you on, but few can help you change like Robyn Downs. So many of us know the type of life we want—happy, fulfilled— but the hard part isn't always the *what*, it's the *how*. With warmth, vulnerability, and stunning clarity, Downs upends our notions of what it means to be and do well, and offers actionable advice for anyone who is ready to change their mindset, and with it, their lives."

—ALICIA MENENDEZ, author of *The Likeability Trap*

"This book will set you free. *The Feel Good Effect* is a breath of much needed fresh air in the self-development space. Robyn graciously and effectively guides you away from a cookie-cutter mindset regarding feeling good, and toward embodying methodologies and paths unique to who you are. Robyn has created a beautiful roadmap to help us thrive forward."

—LALAH DELIA, spiritual writer, wellness educator, and author of *Vibrate Higher Daily*

"This book is straight-up refreshing, inspiring, and so tangible in its advice for living a better life. It's made up of equal parts science-backed research and Robyn's personal stories that will have you simultaneously laughing, crying, nodding, and feeling like someone is finally reading your mind. *The Feel Good Effect* is a must-read for any high-achiever who is craving more peace and joy, as well as a more sustainably healthy way to live. It takes wellness to a whole new (and needed) level."

—SARAH ADLER, founder of Simply Real Health

THE
FEEL
GOOD
EFFECT

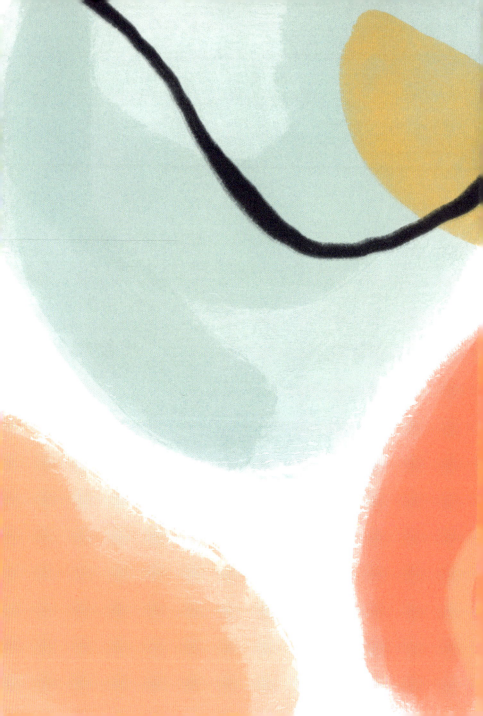

THE

FEEL

GOOD

EFFECT

Reclaim Your Wellness by Finding
Small Shifts That Create Big Change

ROBYN CONLEY DOWNS

ILLUSTRATIONS BY BRIANA SUMMERS

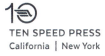

TEN SPEED PRESS
California | New York

To Andrew and Elle.

This is all because of you.

This is all for you.

Library of Congress Cataloging-in-Publication Data

Names: Downs, Robyn Conley, 1980- author.
Title: The feel good effect : how small shifts in thinking create big changes
    / Robyn Conley Downs ; illustrations by Briana Summers.
Description: [Emeryville], California : Ten Speed Press, [2020] |
    Includes index.
Identifiers: LCCN 2020003796 (print) | LCCN 2020003797 (ebook)
    ISBN 9781984858245 (hardcover) | ISBN 9781984858252 (ebook)
Subjects: LCSH: Change (Psychology) | Attitude (Psychology) | Habit. |
    Well-being.
Classification: LCC BF637.C4 D69 2020 (ebook) | LCC BF637.C4 (print) |
    DDC 158.1--dc23
LC record available at https://lccn.loc.gov/2020003796
LC record available at https://lccn.loc.gov/2020003797

Hardcover ISBN: 978-1-9848-5824-5
eBook ISBN: 978-1-9848-5825-2

Printed in China

Design by Annie Marino

10 9 8 7 6 5 4 3 2 1

First Edition

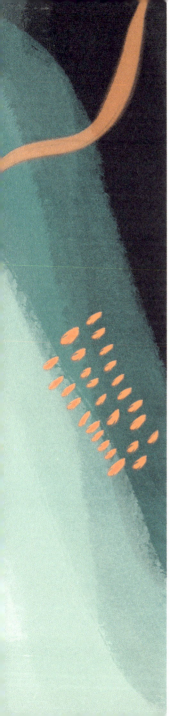

Contents

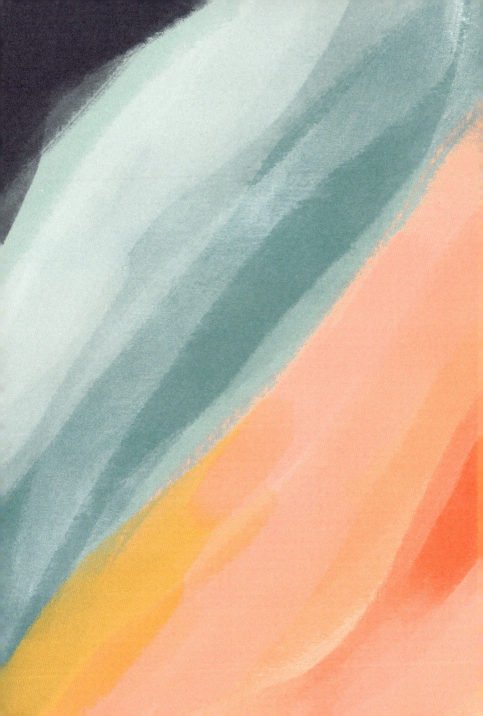

Introduction

Seven months after my daughter, Elle, was born, I stood in the middle of our living room in tears. And I'm not talking a few tears that could easily be brushed away. I'm talking a full-out epic kind of meltdown. The morning had started predictably enough. Waking up early, rushing to feed myself and Elle, frantically getting ready, throwing everything together for the day, trying to get out the door. But right before I was about to leave, my husband, Andrew, asked me what time I planned to be home from work. Seems like an innocent enough question; right? Wrong.

To me, at that particular moment in life, seven months postpartum and trying desperately to figure out a new normal, that small question triggered something much bigger. The problem was, I wasn't actually sure when I'd be home. Beyond that, I couldn't see how I was going to handle all the responsibilities piled up on my to-do list for the day. And I didn't know how I was going to find even one spare minute to take care of myself. Everything felt heavy. At that moment I wondered: How had my life become so complicated, so difficult to navigate? When had taking care of myself become such a low priority?

What's more, I wasn't exactly sure how I'd arrived at this point. Clearly adding a tiny human to the mix wasn't making things easier, but these feelings had deep roots, going back years into my past. To be honest, I had a history of always adding more to my plate, without ever taking anything away. I was a pusher, and I had a tendency to ignore my health and happiness in pursuit of achievement and success. I was striving to have it all even though I didn't have a clear sense of what "having it all" actually meant. And I never stopped to ask myself how I felt, because my mental and physical health seemed irrelevant and not something I had time to prioritize.

HOW TO (NOT) FEEL GOOD

The truth is I'd been teetering for years—advancing up the corporate ladder, attending school on nights and weekends, logging countless hours in front of a computer; all of which had taken a huge toll on both my health and happiness. My motto had always been "just push through," yet even as I strived to do *all the things*, I frequently felt like I wasn't making any progress. Yes, I was grateful for all the gifts in my life, but despite my good fortune I felt a crippling sense that nothing was good enough. Lying in bed at night I'd run through a mental list of things not yet accomplished, and in the morning I'd wake up with a general sense of already being behind.

On that sunny September morning the real reason for my breakdown was that I was convinced the problem was with *me*. That I just needed to find more willpower, to be a little more motivated, to really get my act together. I blamed my struggles not on how I was structuring and approaching my life but rather on my obvious lack of self-control. It seemed there were only two options: go all-in on everything—job, friendships, relationships, and a litany of life responsibilities—or just give up altogether. And at that moment, the giving-up option looked pretty appealing.

Plus I felt like I was the only one struggling, the only one who couldn't figure it out. Looking around at other people's lives, I could list two dozen ways I felt I wasn't measuring up. All my friends seemed to have it more together than I did. They seemed to balance work and family and taking care of themselves with such ease. Why couldn't I do the same? I wanted desperately to figure out how they were doing it. In truth, I wanted my own slice of that magical/perfect/healthy life.

You know the one I'm talking about. The one with an hour-long morning routine (not including meditation) and a perfectly composed organic smoothie. The one with incredibly productive workweeks in which everything on the to-do list gets done. The one with six-pack abs resulting from a seven-day-a-week workout routine—including cardio, stretching, high-intensity strength training, *and* deeply restorative yoga. The one with every meal planned, and everything prepped ahead, all cooked from scratch. The one where I had time to spare for deep breathing, and no screens, and plenty of sleep, and reading, and time with the family. The one where I never had a negative thought.

Eventually, I pulled myself together that morning in the living room, resigned to another long commute, got in the car, and drove to work. Stuck in traffic on the way, I couldn't shake the feeling that something had to give. As I continued to reflect on my situation, I knew things had to change, knew *I* needed to change. As I eventually pulled into my parking spot at work, I knew that I couldn't continue down the path I was on, that it simply wasn't sustainable for myself, or for my family. At that moment in the parking lot that September, I vowed to make a change. The only problem? I had no idea where to start. "If I knew what to do," I thought to myself, "wouldn't I already be doing it?"

GO BIG OR GO HOME

As the days passed, I continued to think about my conundrum, and I began to formulate a plan. And then I decided to do what I always did. I committed to go big. The week following that living room meltdown

I vowed to make big, drastic, life-altering changes. Determined to find that magical/perfect/healthy life, I promised myself that things were going to change. In my mind this was an all-or-nothing situation, and I wanted it all. So with every ounce of the motivation I could pull together, I threw myself into every wellness fad and trend *like it was my job*.

Ignoring the fact that I already had a full-time job and a family, I crammed 60-minute daily workouts into my currently packed schedule. I gave up entire food groups, jumping from diet to diet, convinced that eventually I'd find the perfect one. I spent Sundays planning meals and prepping the daylight hours away. I made pages of lists and checked every box. I bought all the productivity planners, spending more hours than I'd like to admit coming up with elaborate, color-coded outlines to fit everything in. I pushed through. I disciplined. I martialed my willpower. I forced myself to think positively, and I felt guilty when I wasn't able to constantly do so. When things didn't go as planned, and I felt like I'd fallen off the wagon, I'd mentally beat myself up until I got back on track.

And do you know what happened?

It worked.

That go-big-or-go-home approach got results. As in fantastic, absolutely exhilarating, totally amazing *short-term* results. I know, I know—you probably thought I was going to tell you that it didn't work. But that's not the truth. After going to extremes, I got the kind of outward results that had friends stopping me on the street to ask what I was doing. All of a sudden I was a success story, a real-life embodiment of the coveted "after" picture.

Everyone wanted to know what had changed, what was my big secret? Because that's the thing about extremes, deprivation, and willpower—they can work really well for a short period of time. My new way of eating had cleared up my skin, and my body felt lighter. The strenuous workout regimen had made me stronger too. True, my energy was zapped by the end of the day, and I still felt behind and mildly frantic most of the time, but I didn't care. This was working! I was doing it!

But even though my body was changing physically, my mind was still stuck in the same old thought patterns. *What is wrong with you? Is this the best you can do? Really? Can't you get it together for good? Everyone else seems to be able to figure this out, so why can't you?*

The ugly truth was that even though I was achieving what appeared to be success on the outside, my mindset was causing me to feel bad even when I should have been feeling good. I'd hit a goal, but I couldn't stop to appreciate the moment because I was constantly focused on the future. Addicted to the short-term results, I found myself desperately seeking the next best thing, and becoming frustrated when results started to plateau. Still stuck in the comparison game, I found it difficult to stop using other people as a measure of my own success. I was striving and pushing, looking around at what everyone else was doing and then panicking because my results were starting to seem unsustainable. How could I possibly keep up with it all? Plus I had the sneaking suspicion that my new approach was causing me to miss the beautiful life I had right in front of me.

Simply put, the more I strived, the worse I felt. The unrealistic standards, the go-big-or-go-home approach, the everyone-else-can-so-why-can't-I dichotomy? It all started to catch up with me. And then it caught up with me in a big way. Unable to keep up with the impossible, overly complicated situation I'd created, I started to fall behind. Having no way of dealing with setbacks, every upset in my routine, every work trip, and every unplanned illness threw me completely off my game. It was a roller coaster of ups and downs, and I had no idea how to deal with it. I'd tapped my discipline and drained my willpower and, without solid routines and habits to fall back on, I struggled to keep up.

Eventually those short-term results—the ones to which I'd become so attached—all started to evaporate. Tired of feeling deprived, I gave up on healthful eating. Burned out on hours at the gym and marathon meal-prep sessions, I abruptly quit both. Exhausted with productivity for productivity's sake, I abandoned my complicated color-coded schedule. And falling back on old familiar habits, I found myself back in the loop of beating myself up for not being able to follow through. Only this time it was worse because I now had solid proof that I was incapable of sticking with anything. That's the problem with short-term results. By definition, they can't last. I didn't have a problem with motivation. I had a problem with consistency and commitment.

DOUGHNUTS AND STICKER CHARTS

I remember the exact moment when everything started to unravel. I had committed to one of those 30-day challenges at my gym. You know what I'm talking about, the one in which you earn a sticker for each day of completed workouts. The problem was, I'd committed to the challenge without checking to see if I had the right supports in place in my life to facilitate actually completing the challenge.

Things went fine for the first week, and I remember feeling so satisfied with my perfect line of uninterrupted stickers, each representing a day's completed workout. But then, somewhere around day 12, I missed a day. "No big deal," I told myself, "I've still got this." I missed the next day, too, and then the following day. Three days missed. Three missing stickers. And for some reason, knowing there was this gap in my progress, such an obvious indicator of failure, set off a chain of events that changed my life forever.

Stirred up by the sticker failure I decided that, instead of just going back to the gym and picking up where I left off, the best course of action would be to quit the challenge altogether. Since I'd clearly messed it up, I might as well give up. Not only that, instead of figuring out an alternative workout for the day, I decided to head to the doughnut place on the way home. I know; right? Now, hear me out. There's absolutely nothing wrong with eating a doughnut. But for me, on that day, the doughnut represented a white flag. Sinking my teeth into the warm, glazed gooeyness, I decided I was done. Like really freaking *done*.

I felt like I was out of options, and at that point I felt like I'd tried *all* the options, following every piece of conventional wisdom and advice to the letter. Thinking positively? You betcha. Setting SMART goals? Check. Discipline and willpower? Double check. Juice fasting, step counting, meal planning, downloading *alllllll* the mindfulness apps? Check, check, double check. Comparing myself to everyone else and trying to do it all? One hundred percent, check. Feeling broken down and frustrated, I was out of motivation and ideas. Sitting there in the dimly lit pastry shop, rain streaming down the windows, I wondered why something as seemingly innocent as a sticker chart had sent me into such a tailspin. Maybe it was the doughnut sugar rush, or the soft glow of the shop's fluorescent sign, but at that moment I began to feel something very small shift within me. No, this wasn't a huge eureka moment, nor a triumphant aha, but rather a very subtle shift in thinking.

At that moment I began to wonder if perhaps I'd been looking at the problem all wrong. As I pondered this thought, more questions sprang to mind. Questions like "Does this really have to be so hard?" and "Is the pursuit of wellness actually making me well?" and "Is this really what I want my life to look like?" and finally, "What does it really mean to be healthy and happy anyway?" Finishing my doughnut and heading home, I felt strangely optimistic. As Andrew and I sat down to eat dinner that night, I shared the story of my day. After downloading all the sticker-chart and doughnut details, he and I fell into a discussion about what it really means to be happy and healthy.

WHAT IT REALLY MEANS TO BE HEALTHY

When I stopped to think about the definitions of *happy* and *healthy*, it seemed strange that while these words are used so frequently, it's difficult to pinpoint what they actually mean. Similarly, it seemed that if I didn't know what they meant, it was going to be hard to accomplish either. After a long discussion, Andrew eventually concluded our conversation by saying, "I think at the end of the day, health and happiness are really about feeling good." "Hmmmmm," I thought. "Could it be that simple?"

Of course, the term *feel good* can be defined in a number of different ways, and it's possible to think of it as instant gratification, hedonism, or the superficial high of outward validation. But that's not how I was thinking about it then, nor is it how I define it now. I'll say more about how I define *feeling good* in "Feel Good Fallacy" on page 17, but at that moment around the dinner table, I began to think of "feeling good" as an overall sense of well-being in mind, body, and soul. According to this definition, at that point in my life, I was most definitely *not* feeling good.

I assume if you picked up this book, you can relate on some level. I'm sure your specific story is different from mine, but some of those attempts at striving, pushing through, the on-again-off-again routine, or getting caught in the comparison trap may strike a chord. Perhaps, like me, you've at times felt exhausted by the do's and don'ts. Don't eat this. Do eat that. Exercise this way. But not that way. Do better. Go bigger. Find more hours in the day. Figure out how to do it all, and do it all perfectly. Or maybe, like me, you've experienced short-term results, only to fall back into old habits. The gym membership sits unused. The drive-through line beckons you back. You write a few pages and then give up on the entire project. Or perhaps, you've had times when you've beaten yourself up for not getting it all right, or telling yourself you need to be a more motivated, disciplined person to get the results you're looking for.

Perhaps you've felt crushed by business, like you're not doing enough, or you've felt guilty, burned out, or out of balance. Or maybe you're concerned that if you continue down the path you're on, pushing and striving, that eventually your health and happiness are going to suffer. Maybe you've felt like there's always *more*—more to do, more to be, more to have. And perhaps you feel there must be a better way, though you're unsure of exactly how to make the change.

If you've ever felt this way, or if you feel this way right this minute, I want you to know you are not alone. I get it. *I have been there.* That striving, pushing, comparing, the starting and stopping? I've lived all of it. That approach used to be my baseline, my lifeline, and the only way I knew. So if you feel like you're working harder, not smarter; if you're running on the hamster wheel of comparison; or if you feel like you can't finish what you start? I see you. If you're so stressed and exhausted at the end of the day that the only option seems like a giant glass of wine and a Netflix binge? I understand. Or if you struggle to make good habits stick, to find consistency, and to actually feel good in the process, well, you're not alone in that either. I was you. But here's what I want you to know.

You are not failing. You are not a failure.

Seriously, let that sink in. And as it turns out, neither was I. Eventually, when I finally paused to ask myself the basic question, *What about actually feeling good?* I realized that maybe I wasn't the problem after all. Following the small mental shift that occurred in the dough-nut shop, and the conversation with Andrew, I came to the conclusion that maybe my approach was failing me. Perhaps the conventional wisdom and advice I was following was wrong in the first place. And maybe, just maybe, I didn't need to start over—*again*.

Following the dinner with Andrew, I found myself tossing and turn-ing in bed, unable to shut off my mind and fall asleep. As my family slept, I crept downstairs, flipped on a light, lit a fire, and settled in with a notebook, pencil, and a pure, stubborn determination to figure out a better way. At the time I didn't know exactly what that would mean, but I did know it could not be more of the same. I had a strong sense that what was required was a fundamental shift in the way I was approaching the problem. As I paused to reflect, I also knew that I needed to start trusting myself and that this time working harder was not going to be the answer. As the flames flickered, I committed right then and there to step out of my old way of doing things and into a simpler, more consistent, flat-out joyful way to be. I committed to making feeling good not just the end goal but also the process along the way.

On that sleepless night, I began to imagine a way out of striving and struggling and a way in to lasting, consistent change. I knew, too, that this change was going to take time, and many small shifts. I felt a strong pull to actually enjoy the process, rather than sacrifice my life to meet arbitrary goals. And I knew that to do all this I'd need to let go of some things in order to make room for more calm, more focus, and more ease. That night, in my living room, I decided to stop chasing "perfect" and instead embrace "gentle." I decided it was finally time. It was time to feel good.

And you know what? I believe it's your time too.

THE FEEL GOOD EFFECT

When I finally came to my realization—that I wasn't the problem, that maybe it was my approach that was broken—it gave me a new place to start. Because here's the thing I haven't mentioned up until now. At the time of that meltdown in my living room—that morning in September—I was actually enrolled in a doctoral program studying decision-making theory (i.e., how people make decisions) and public health policy (i.e., how to make maintaining health easier as well as more accessible).

Before that, I'd earned a master's degree in education and behavior change, focusing on teaching people how to form new healthful habits and behaviors. Also, Andrew, my partner in research and in life, is a clinical psychologist with a PhD in behavior change. Between the two of us, we've spent more than five decades studying how the brain works, how people make decisions, and how to create health habits. After years of studying and researching, you'd think that I would be putting these teachings into practice in my own life. But I wasn't.

That's the thing; technically I knew what to do, I just wasn't doing it. Basically, I was failing to apply what I knew in theory to the reality of my own life. At the time, I was also studying systems thinking, or how parts of a system work together to create a cohesive whole. It was thinking about systems that finally allowed everything to click for me.

What I realized is that I didn't have an effective system for my own life to support the results I was seeking, nor did I have a system that allowed all the parts of my life to work together efficiently. I began to think that perhaps the best course of action would be to use my professional background to figure out a better solution. A solution that would take into account how the brain works, how we make decisions and form habits, and, ultimately, how all these things work together in the context of real life to support the results we're after.

A DIFFERENT APPROACH

After that late night on the couch in front of the fire, I began to formulate a plan. This time, though, my plan was different from what I'd tried before. I committed to read everything I could get my hands on, listen to all the podcasts, and dive into the research on my own. If it had to do with how the brain works, behavior change, habits, mindset, routines, goal setting, or mindfulness, I was on it.

In the process, I began to find a wealth of valuable information, plus some stuff that, frankly, seemed out of touch. Reading the recommendations, I had to wonder, did these people have real lives? Did they have 9-to-5 jobs, long commutes, difficult coworkers, or challenging bosses? Did any of them deal with dropping kids off at school, doing chores, making appointments, or the litany of daily life tasks that interfere with their recommendations? It didn't seem like it.

In short, many of the recommendations, particularly those I came across in popular media, appeared to be written for someone living in a perfect world, while I was living in the *real* world. I had a job and a commute; I attended school at night; and I didn't have a full-time nanny, a personal assistant, or a live-in housecleaner. Dissatisfied with many of the recommendations, I realized that I was going to have to figure out a set of solutions that worked for me, in real life.

I continued down the research rabbit hole, tapping into the science on how the brain works, how to be consistent with goals, and how to make habits stick and be sustainable. Partnering with Andrew on the research-method side of things, I developed a framework that I then started to test in my own life. As I tested and tweaked, running countless small experiments, I started to notice something—specifically, a pattern of assumptions that I had been making through all those years of trying to create change in my life. Looking at assumptions—or ideas believed to be true—is something I'd learned to do in my policy program. That is, whenever setting out to solve a big policy program, I'd learned that the best place to start is by looking at assumptions and then asking a simple question: Are these true?

Soon, I found myself writing a short list of the assumptions I'd previously thought to be true in my quest for health and happiness. Here's what I came up with at the time.

FALSE ASSUMPTIONS ABOUT HOW TO GET RESULTS AND LASTING CHANGE

- You should make drastic changes and big shifts, usually all at once.

- You need to be a disciplined, motivated person.

- You must have a lot of willpower.

- You should deprive yourself.

- You need to focus only on habits.

- You must set incredibly high standards and be hard on yourself if you don't achieve them.

- Success is best measured externally, by comparison to other people, and in a binary way—either you succeed, or you don't.

Once I had this list of assumptions, I continued to test my framework and study the research. One thing became very clear: All this time I had been going about change backward, focusing on the wrong things and using faulty assumptions. I thought that results require one set of things, when they really require something very different.

These realizations led me to ask a completely new series of questions. Questions such as, "What if results don't require drastic change, an overreliance on willpower, or excessive discipline?" "What if change comes from managing the way we think, and the way we structure our days?" and, "What if success can be measured differently, and can come from a set of skills that can be learned rather than something we're born with?"

From this new place of understanding, I began the work of creating an approach that would allow success to be measured differently. My aim was to rely on research-based practices to support the process of change in real life. I wanted to develop a set of practices and systems that would facilitate working smarter, not harder, and to embody a *gentle is the new perfect* approach, a simple mantra that has since become my motto, and my mission. Over time, I began to synthesize the work into both a mindset (the ingrained thought patterns that influence actions and results) and a method (a system of strategies and habits that support change). Along the way I also started a website, Real Food Whole Life, and a podcast, the Feel Good Effect, with the intent to share what I was learning. As I shared this content, I began to receive countless emails and messages from readers and listeners who were experiencing profound effects when using the approach in their own lives. Over and over I'd hear stories of transformation, of people finding the life-changing effects that come from small shifts in mindset and methods.

Today my life feels drastically different from that September morning in my living room, and from waving the white flag at the doughnut shop. It's important to point out here, too, that while my life *feels* different, it's not actually all that different day to day. I still work full time as I did back then, and I still value eating well, moving my body regularly, and taking care of my mind. My life is still full of responsibilities, appointments, work, friends, and family. I haven't opted out, quit my job, thrown out my phone, or moved off the grid. When it seems like so much of the wellness advice these days is to quit everything or change your life completely, I've gone the other direction. I didn't stop everything, and you don't have to either.

Instead of opting out, I've evolved my approach. This has occurred by way of small changes in thinking and action, which has allowed me to streamline my responsibility-laden life using a system that allows for more ease. The constant ups and downs no longer shake me, and I trust myself, knowing that my life isn't going to look like anyone else's. It's this uniqueness that makes my life beautiful. Accepting this uniqueness, and the ups and downs that come with it, is what makes my life mine.

This is the Feel Good Effect, a positive change resulting from shifts in mindset and daily actions. The Feel Good Effect is an approach to life, a mindset and a method that work together to harness the power of your brain, to create small shifts in thinking, to find commitment and consistency, and to create a system of strategies and habits that work to get you results. And while it's an approach that offers radical results, the process itself is not radical. Incredibly practical, ultra-sane, and completely effective, it's designed to get results in the context of real life, without deprivation or suffering for the process.

THE FEEL GOOD MINDSET AND THE GOOD METHOD

The Feel Good Effect begins with the Feel Good Mindset, a powerful way of thinking based on neuroscience, positive psychology, human development, and mindfulness. This mindset will allow you to shift the way you think so you can enjoy the process of change, be more resilient, and experience real, lasting success.

Next up, the GOOD Method is a simple system of strategies and habits designed to get you the results you want, without working so hard for them. The GOOD Method is effective in part because it targets daily habits, which account for about *45 percent of your behavior* in any given day, plus the life routines in which those habits exist.

MINDSET + METHOD =

feel good effect

It's the combination of the mindset and the method that work synergistically to create the Feel Good Effect, producing positive changes in your patterns of thinking and daily actions. The Feel Good Effect creates a powerful upward spiral that will allow you to get lasting results, create sustainable habits, make better decisions, and feel good in your life right now. More than just theory, the Feel Good Mindset gives you specific practices to allow you to shift your thoughts and behaviors. And more than just a list of habits, the GOOD Method pulls together science-based strategies into a practical system designed to work in real life.

Don't worry, though, if research isn't your thing; you don't need a special degree or to love science for the Feel Good Effect to work. That's the beauty of the approach—so much of the work has already been done for you. Of course, if you do want details on specific studies and research mentioned in this book, you can find a list of references at realfoodwholelife.com/fgebook.

All that's required here is an open mind, a willingness to make small changes, and an adoption of new practices. To know that this isn't about trying to change who you are as a person. The work of this book in many ways is the opposite; it's about more deeply connecting with yourself. This isn't about ignoring the challenges in your life or asking you to stifle your emotions. The Feel Good Effect doesn't require you to be happy all the time, to never have a negative thought, to opt out of everything, or to flip your life upside down all at once. Instead, the work requires an openness to the idea that change is possible and a letting go of old ways of thinking and actions that no longer serve you. True success will come through trusting the process and yourself, and allowing time to work its magic. You just need to show up. Make small shifts. See how everything changes. This might also require a little permission. Permission to do things differently. To let it be easy and joyful. To know that your success isn't going to look like someone else's and that self-kindness is the pathway to the results you're seeking. Permission to know that you deserve this.

Because you deserve to feel good.

One of the best parts about this approach is that you can start right now. There's no need to wait for January, or Monday, for the kids to leave home, to quit your job, or to go back to school. You can start at this very moment, even if your life is full of challenges, setbacks, or difficulties. You can start right here, right now, by taking tiny, incremental steps. You can start where you are, take your time, and go at your own pace. Know, too, that there is no better moment than right now to show up for your life. Know that you're ready, qualified, and completely capable of taking action. Know that together we will reframe what success looks like. This book will show you how.

USING THIS BOOK

You hold in your hands a step-by-step guide to creating the Feel Good Effect in your own life. All the information is available to you now, and my hope is that this book will also serve as a lifelong blueprint, one filled with resources you can return to whenever you need, as often as you like. Here are a few things to keep in mind in order to get the most out of this book.

FEEL GOOD FALLACY

Occasionally, when I explain the Feel Good Effect, I come across someone who gets hung up on the term "feel good," confusing it with taking the easy route, being selfish, or going for immediate gratification. To be clear, feeling good is none of those things. Feeling good doesn't mean you disregard other people's needs, that you feel happy all the time, or that you ignore the serious problems of the world. Feeling good doesn't mean everything is easy, either. Instead, as you'll see, feeling good is something you will define for yourself. It can be generally defined as a feeling of ease, well-being, meaning, and fulfillment.

A DIFFERENT KIND OF OPTIMIZATION

Plenty of books already exist about mindset, habits, and routines, and they are often presented as a means to accomplish more. Their point is to optimize for more—more time for the sake of more time, or more productivity for the sake of more productivity. This book is different. It's about optimizing and maximizing for feeling good. Feeling good, then, is both the end goal *and* a means to get there. Wild, I know. Of course, the process outlined in the book will allow more time for what matters, for you to be more strategically productive, and to create space for meaning. But still, one of the primary goals of this book is to help you optimize differently, and that is to optimize feeling good.

RADICAL CONSISTENCY AND COMMITMENT

I've found that some people, at first, can be attached to the idea that discipline, willpower, and motivation are the keys to success, and to the idea that *consistency* is the same thing as *perfection*. If this describes you, I invite you to read with an open mind, as this book offers an alternative, research-based approach showing that real, lasting results are instead possible through the practice of commitment and consistency, implemented imperfectly and incrementally over time.

TEAM TINY CHANGES

Occasionally on my podcast, the Feel Good Effect, I invite my audience to join me on "team tiny changes." My intention is to remind my listeners of the power of the small and incremental. In this book, I invite you to do the same, take what you need and leave what you don't, one of my favorite sayings, borrowed from the yoga community. Let both serve as simple reminders that small changes count just as much as big ones, and that you are always welcome to take what works for you right now and to leave the rest.

REFRAME YOUR MINDSET

The first section of this book will walk you through mindset, including what it is and why it matters. You'll also discover the Striving Mindset, which will allow you to better understand your brain, including why some of your current thought patterns may not be serving you. Then you'll get the rundown on the Feel Good Mindset, so you can flip the script and rewire your brain. Sprinkled throughout, you'll find specific practical exercises to shift your thinking toward the Feel Good Mindset.

COMMIT TO THE METHOD

The second section is where you'll find the GOOD Method, a system of four strategies and habits designed to support you in getting lasting results. This method is designed to amplify the Feel Good Mindset; as you practice one, the other benefits. Each strategy within the GOOD Method can be used alone, or combined together for an even bigger impact. Each chapter also offers a specific exercise to help you put the method into practice.

UPGRADE YOUR LIFE

In the final section, you'll find an action plan to take the Feel Good Effect beyond the book and into your life, along with a simple challenge designed to help you take action, one small step at a time. The challenge can be completed alone or with others. Accountability goes a long way here, so I encourage you to grab a friend or family member and do the challenge together. You'll find more resources to support you at realfoodwholelife.com/fgebook.

Okay, now we're ready. Let's make it happen!

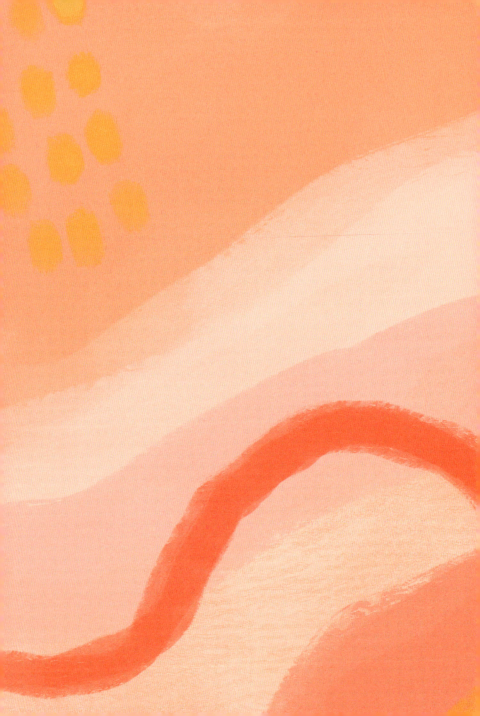

Mindset

ONE

Change Your Brain, Change Your Life

Can I tell you a secret? What got you here, reading this book right now, probably won't take you where you want to go. Before I explain, let's rewind for just a second, back to that moment in the doughnut shop. Up until that point in my life, I thought that the only way to make real change was to focus on things such as finding the perfect app, the exact right workout plan, and the elusive diet that I could actually stick to. That was when I measured success according to a list of unrealistic standards I'd created for myself, in reference to what other people were doing, when I thought I needed to somehow become a motivated and disciplined person in order to make forward progress.

WHAT GOT YOU HERE (WON'T TAKE YOU WHERE YOU WANT TO GO)

The thing is, I have always had plenty of motivation; at the start. I'd buy all the right produce at the store, sign up for the gym, download the app. I was practically a professional New Year's resolution maker. But inevitably, no matter how motivated I was at the beginning, life seemed to get in the way. Most of the groceries from my new way of eating would end up in the trash, replaced by a wave of guilt about throwing it away. I'd start off strong, but eventually the gym membership would go unused. And before long, the new mindfulness app would sit ignored, another remnant of things I'd started but couldn't stick with.

If you've ever found yourself in a similar start-slide-stop cycle, know that you're not alone. The truth is, the vast majority of New Year's resolutions fail, gym memberships go unused, and diets get abandoned. The dirty little secret is that motivation *by itself* is simply not enough to sustain long-term change. Sure, that initial burst gets you to sign up for the gym, to download the app, to buy all the groceries, but when it comes to sticking with it over time, it doesn't last. Because in the never-ending search for wellness, we've missed something monumental.

What we're missing is mindset.

THE PROBLEM WITH MOTIVATION,
DISCIPLINE, AND WILLPOWER

Mindset—the *way* you think—is actually what most affects your decisions, actions, and ultimately your results. That's why just trying to be motivated, or disciplined, or have willpower doesn't work long term. In truth, motivation, discipline, and willpower are all mental resources that deplete over time. Alone, they aren't enough to change what you do every day or to get lasting results. A much better use of your time and attention is to focus on the specific skills and actions you need in order to create sustainable change. These will allow you to be committed and consistent.

The tricky thing about mindset is it's . . . well, invisible. It's a sneaky saboteur, so ingrained that it can keep you stuck and feeling terrible for years. It's probably the real reason you're not getting results. In truth, the way you think—your ingrained thought patterns—make a huge difference in how you live, affecting everything from your ability to be resilient and adopt new strategies to the formation of new habits and making daily decisions, all of which impact your results.

The reason we often miss mindset is that it happens behind the scenes *inside* the brain, something you don't notice until you start paying attention to it. So even though mindset is the foundation upon which change is built—the thing that actually matters most—we most often skip it in favor of trying to adopt a new habit, set a new goal, or muster up motivation. But skipping mindset is going about the problem backward. Without a solid foundation in place, it's far more likely that you'll end up in that familiar start-slide-stop cycle, thinking that you're not doing your part.

Skipping mindset can have you feeling completely frustrated because the new workout habit didn't stick (again), burning out at work because you can't seem to keep up, beating yourself up because of the all-out weekend pizza binge, or striving to do it all instead of being present in your own life. You keep telling yourself that if you just work harder, set better habits, find the perfect plan, or follow the latest workout trend to the letter, then things will be different. That *you* will be different. The good news? It doesn't have to be this way.

In this chapter I'm going to break down exactly how mindset works, so you can untangle ineffective patterns and find a better way. Understanding mindset, and managing that incredible mind of yours, will give you the keys to unlock the results you're seeking, putting an end to the cycle of striving. This is the first step, understanding what's really going on and opening up to the possibility of another way.

That's why we're starting here, instead of skipping ahead to routines, strategies, and habits. Because without mindset, none of the other stuff will work in the long term. So let's start at the beginning. You can absolutely do this, and you can do it on your own terms. You just need to find a new way that sticks and is sustainable. For you.

THE POWER OF MINDSET

Mindset is one of those words that are popping up just about everywhere these days, but it's used in so many different ways it's hard to figure out what it actually means. While it might seem as if mindset is the new cure-all—"Good Vibes Only!" "Think Positive Thoughts!" "Ten Ways to Have a More Uplifting Mindset!"—I honestly cringe a little when I see stuff like this pop up on my social-media feeds. Mindset is about *so much more* than thinking positively, manifesting, or mantras. The problem with the mindset-equals-positivity trend is that it ignores the complexity of the human brain, implying that if you're not getting the results you want, it's somehow your fault for not thinking positively enough.

Because if you really were thinking positively, you'd be getting results; right? Want to lose weight? Think positively! Trying to grow your family? Make sure you're thinking positively! Want a college degree?

Gotta think positively! Looking for success at work? Positivity, baby! And if those things haven't happened for you? Well, then, you aren't thinking positively *enough*. But what happens if you're trying to think positively, have a bad day, and end up thinking a negative thought? Not only are you neglecting to think positively but you're also beating yourself up because of it. And the cycle continues.

Now, I'm definitely not saying to ditch positivity; I'm just saying that "positive thinking" and "manifesting" are not the same as *mindset*. I'm also saying that you don't have to think positively all the time, or stifle the full spectrum of your feelings and emotions in order to get results. You can still have bad days, experience moments of self-doubt, and have life setbacks. Heck, you can even think negative thoughts sometimes. I know; right?!

Because mindset is about something more. That amazing brain of yours is one powerful part of you, so talking about mindset means we're going to get in there and think about thinking. Meta, but stick with me. Like I said, mindset is not the thought itself, trying to control your thoughts, or trying to think only happy thoughts. It's not forcing yourself to work harder all the time or to be someone you're not. Mindset is the actual *way* you think—the ingrained thought patterns that you may not even be aware of because they're basically automatic. And these ingrained thought patterns? They affect everything from how you process information to how you form habits to how you make decisions. All of this together then affects how you act and behave, and the end results. Mindset is a seriously powerful thing.

MINDSET DEFINED

The concept of mindset used to seem really fuzzy to me. I knew there had to be a reason I was trying so hard but not seeing results. When I tapped in to the neuroscience and psychology on how the brain works, though, it became clear just how important mindset is. Yet I still struggled to define it. It seemed the term was being used in so many different ways that I had a hard time understanding what it meant. After digging into the research, though, I was able to create a simple definition.

What we think of as *mindset* is essentially a set of recurring thought-pattern loops inside our brains. This super-dynamic set of patterns creates a chain reaction that influences our everyday actions and eventually our results too. I call this set of reactions the Mindset Loop. The Mindset Loop happens over and over, day in and day out, and, over time, the reaction reinforces itself to the point where it becomes so automatic that we often don't notice it's happening.

The Mindset Loop happens in four distinct steps. Here's how it works.

1   You take in information or you have an experience.

    Let's say, for example, that the experience is skipping a workout.

2   This experience triggers an existing thought pattern in your brain. While there are an infinite number of possible thought patterns, to keep things simple, we'll use just two examples.

    First possible thought pattern: "Ugh, I missed a workout. I totally blew it."

    Second possible thought pattern: "Life got busy; no big deal."

    These two possible thought patterns represent a virtual fork in the road. Although the same experience has occurred (missing a workout), the thought patterns are completely different.

3   Because the thought patterns are different, they trigger different actions.

For example, the first thought pattern—"Ugh, I missed a workout. I totally blew it"—triggers the action of skipping the next day's workout because the options seem binary; either all-in or all-out.

The second thought pattern—"Life got busy; no big deal"—triggers an action of choosing a shorter workout for the next day, because you know there are many options for forward progress.

4 The action triggers a result.

In reality, the result is actually the last step in the Mindset Loop, and with which you are most likely familiar. Since results are what we all want, it's what we tend to over-focus on.

mindset loop

INFORMATION
or
EXPERIENCE

brain interprets
according to
thought pattern

result!

ACTION

In the first example, the action of skipping multiple workouts triggers a specific result: An inconsistent approach to exercise.

Alternatively, in the second example, the action of evaluating realistic options and choosing shorter workouts triggers another result: A consistent approach to exercise.

These Mindset Loops repeat over and over, moment after moment, day after day, adding up to a constellation of results that make up your life. Eventually, results start to influence the way you take in information and the specific experiences you choose to participate in, creating a complete loop.

So simple, yet so completely powerful.

Practicing Mindset Loops makes them become automatic, eventually shaping your life. This is why mindset is such a big deal. While the *only* thing that happened in Step 1 was missing a workout, the outcomes are completely different. One experience, two entirely different results.

MANAGE YOUR MINDSET

As I mentioned, the Mindset Loop becomes automatic pretty quickly, because during that second step—where you interpret an experience according to an existing thought pattern—an actual pathway develops in your brain. And as that pathway develops and is repeated, it becomes ingrained, which means it literally *changes the way your brain is wired*. Those well-worn thought patterns become an actual part of you—so much so that you often don't notice them. That's why your actions, habits, and results can all start to look similar. And even though the possible pathways are infinite, your brain ends up following a similar path each time, because it's become the path of least resistance, leading you right back to the results you get most often.

What you practice, you get better at.

But here's the cool thing about the brain. It can change. Have you ever heard the saying "Neurons that fire together, wire together?" That's called neuroplasticity, meaning that neural pathways form when neurons work together in the same way over time, creating lasting patterns in your brain. Once those pathways form, they become very efficient and automatic, explaining why you might keep getting the same results. The good news about neuroplasticity, though, is that those pathways aren't fixed. As in, you can change them. They aren't stuck.

And neither are you.

By mastering the Mindset Loop, you can change your brain and learn how to manage your mindset. This will shift not just the way you think but also your actions and results. Of course, this isn't a quick fix. If you've spent years practicing one set of thought patterns, shifting to a new way of thinking is not going to happen overnight. But, again, the thing about neuroplasticity is that your brain *can* change, regardless of how long you've practiced old thought patterns. You absolutely don't have to repeat the same old patterns, working hard, and not getting results. So that's exactly what we're going to do, talk about the secret mindset saboteur that might be the biggest barrier to results. It's time to talk about striving.

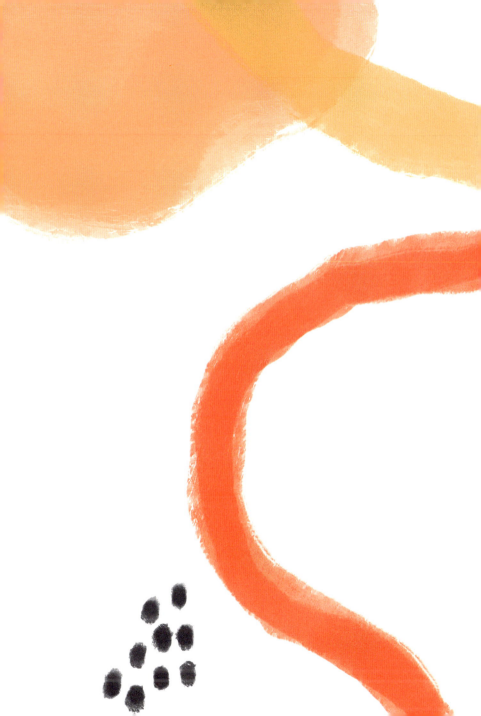

TWO

The Striving Mindset

Have you ever tossed and turned in bed at night, mind racing, feeling like the day passed in a blur of business, yet somehow feeling like you have nothing to show for it? Or have you ever wanted to try something new—a way of eating, a workout, a project at work—but felt paralyzed because you couldn't figure out where to begin, couldn't seem to get it all right from the start? Or maybe you feel it's hard to stop and celebrate small wins in life because, no matter what you do, there's always something more, someone doing it better, or another milestone to achieve? Perhaps life feels like it's zooming past, and you can't seem to pause long enough to enjoy it.

While these scenarios may seem quite different from one another, they all have one thing in common: they all describe *striving*. Striving is so pervasive, such an ingrained part of Western culture, that we often can't even see it. We celebrate and revere people who strive, people for whom *good enough* is never good enough. The athlete who sacrifices everything in the pursuit of greatness. The CEO who works all hours day and night, going without sleep, food, or rest to rise to the top. Go big or go home; take it all; do it better than everyone else. We strive to strive. It's as simple as that.

Striving became second nature to me with high school sports and continued into college, my corporate career, and, eventually, motherhood. A sprinkle of perfectionism here, a burst of all-or-nothing there, all nestled together in a pile of comparison—the trifecta of striving always seemed like the only way to achieve success. The interesting thing is that I didn't realize the negative impact it was having on my well-being because I was so rewarded for it. That's the thing about striving. It's celebrated and reinforced, making it difficult to imagine that there is anything wrong with it. We strive because it has become synonymous with success.

But while striving can yield spectacular short-term results, it's not sustainable. Yes, you can push, and sacrifice, and aim for perfect, but eventually it backfires. This is what I finally realized; the approach that had worked my whole life—the perfection chasing, the black-and-white thinking, the comparison game—was no longer working and was, in fact, making everything in my life harder. Since then, I've come to understand my mindset was affecting my actions and my results, and it was not serving my values or goals, or creating the healthy life I actually wanted. I've also come to realize that there is just *one* mindset standing in the way of sustainable, long-term results: the Striving Mindset.

WHAT IS THE STRIVING MINDSET?

The Striving Mindset—that very all-too-familiar straining, struggling approach—is what's actually standing in the way of lasting change and feeling good. Remember the second part of the Mindset Loop, the part where the brain interprets information according to an existing pattern? This is where the Striving Mindset exists; it's made up of three specific ways of thinking.

striving mindset

PERFECTIONISM

ALL-OR-NOTHING THINKING

COMPARISON

Figuring out the Striving Mindset represented a significant moment in my life. *This* was the reason I kept trying, burning out, and not feeling good. So this is where we're starting, with mindset thought patterns. We're starting here not to shame you, blame you, or slap a label on you but rather to allow you to better understand what's really going on. Because when you comprehend what's actually happening, you can begin to rewire for something better. To create small shifts in thinking that will ultimately change your life. Let's start with perfectionism.

PERFECTIONISM

Chances are you've heard the word *perfectionism* plenty of times. Maybe you even think of yourself as a perfectionist. But my guess is that you probably don't. In truth, most of the time we think of a perfectionist as an identity, or a type of person, and that type of person is usually not us. Think about it. What comes to mind when you hear the word *perfectionist*? Maybe it's a super-type-A person with a perfectly clean car, an immaculate desk, and an impeccable wardrobe. Maybe it's your best friend or sibling—that person in your life who always seems to have it all together.

In truth, while perfectionism is often thought of as a personality trait, associated with a specific type of person, the perfectionist stereotype is not what I'm talking about here. I view perfectionism as *a way of thinking*, or ingrained thought patterns, that shows up in a million different ways. And it can be really hard to recognize from the outside. Such thought patterns pop up for most people, regardless of whether they self-identify as perfectionists.

Perfectionist thought patterns often are the opposite of what we expect. For example, someone stuck in perfectionist thought patterns might have a super-messy car. (Because why clean it if you can't do it perfectly?) Or, a perfectionist thought pattern might cause procrastination and avoidance of starting new things. (Because if you don't know how to do it correctly from the start, why even try?)

THE PERFECTION FILTER

Diet. Productivity. Exercise. Parenting. Relationships. Self-love. Regardless of the category or topic we're talking about, perfectionist thought patterns quickly become a source of stress and suffering. Because with perfectionist thought patterns, regardless of what you're trying to do, the process becomes about doing it perfectly, without ever making a mistake. Which, while impossible, does not seem to stop one from trying.

The research on perfectionism is staggeringly clear; it's damaging and completely counterproductive. In fact, perfectionist thought patterns have been shown to cause a lack of growth, leading people to take fewer risks. Also, perfectionist thought patterns suck the joy out of just about anything. As Dr. Brené Brown, a research professor at the University of Houston, says, perfectionism is a completely destructive (and sadly, kind of addictive) way of thinking, leading you to believe that if you can do everything perfectly, you can avoid feelings of shame, judgment, and blame. And the part that makes this way of thinking really insidious is that *perfect doesn't actually exist.* Perfection is a myth, an illusion, an unrealistic set of ideals that are simply not attainable.

Okay, so now you might be thinking, if perfection isn't possible, then why are we so susceptible to it? Well, as it turns out, there's actually a neuroanatomical bias toward perfectionism in our brains. Which basically means that our brains seem to naturally lean toward perfectionist thought patterns. It's kind of a nature *and* nurture thing happening. Studies show that on a neural level, our brains actually appear to be prewired to respond to mistakes and failures. It's called error-related negativity, and people with high levels of perfectionist thought patterns actually show strong bursts of error-related negativity in their cortex when making a mistake. Making a mistake basically creates a shock to the system.

As mistakes start to be associated with these "shocks," research shows that people with perfectionist thought patterns will go out of their way to avoid making mistakes altogether. Thus, they will self-limit their options in the attempt to avoid making mistakes, missing out on opportunities for growth and improvement. Research has also shown that people with perfectionist thought patterns are more likely to notice setbacks or signs of potential impending failure, making them more likely to give up quickly to avoid the sting of making a mistake. This hardwiring may have evolved as a way to help us avoid making serious, life-threatening mistakes, but in our modern lives it's clearly no longer serving us. Additionally, perfectionist thought patterns are common and seem to be on the rise, particularly in Western cultures, researchers say. Why? In our fast-paced world, people are experiencing more demands, expecting more from others, and expecting more from themselves. Here we are, just trying to live our lives, and our brains are basically on a constant search for perfection.

So, if our brains seem to be naturally wired to seek perfection, and this way of thinking appears to be increasing, you'd think that these thought patterns would get results. *But they don't.* Not even by a long shot. That's what makes them so sneaky.

We think *perfect* is the solution, but it's actually the problem.

THE GUILT GAME

Mom guilt. Guilty pleasure. I feel *so* guilty. Ever notice how often guilt creeps into the daily conversation? Here's the truth; what we think of as guilt is often just perfectionist thought patterns in disguise. I call it the Guilt Game. Take the concept of "mom guilt," I feel guilty when I'm at work because I'm not spending quality time with my kids, and I feel guilty when I'm with my kids because I'm not getting work done. I feel guilty when I'm with my kids because I'm not taking care of myself, and I feel guilty when I'm taking care of myself because I'm not taking care of my kids. This all-too-familiar cycle is really just perfectionist ideals masquerading as feelings of guilt.

Good enough is never good enough, and perfectionist thought patterns can rob you of the opportunity to be present in your one, precious life. This is the destruction that perfectionist thought patterns can cause. Thinking that you can do it all, without ever making a mistake, when in reality, there's really only a finite amount of time and attention in the day. Thinking that if you could only figure out a way to get it all done without mistakes or trade-offs—working *and* spending time with your family *and* taking care of yourself *and* taking care of those around you, all at the same time—then you would be happy. This is the trap of perfection. Because mistakes and trade-offs are an inherent part of the human experience.

Of course, in small doses, perfectionist thought patterns can help propel people to greatness, to push hard, and to achieve at high levels. This is why it's such a seductive thought pattern. But research shows that perfectionist thought patterns rarely show up in small doses. Instead, they quickly creep in, infiltrate your daily existence, and eventually backfire.

Take productivity. Perfectionist thought patterns actually have an *adverse* impact on productivity, causing procrastination and risk avoidance. Getting stuck in the perfectionist thinking trap means you're far more likely to procrastinate over the things you know are important, or avoid doing them altogether. Be honest, can you think of a time when you procrastinated over starting something because you didn't know how to get it exactly right at the onset? Or you didn't have the proper game plan, or all the pieces to the puzzle? These are all perfectionist thought patterns. Perfectionism? It's often the root cause of procrastination. Research also links perfectionism with a litany of mental health risks, including cortisol spikes, depression, anxiety, and mood disorders. As in, perfectionist thought patterns are more likely to make you stressed, depressed, and anxious. Essentially, perfectionism makes you miserable, negatively impacts mental health and well-being, *and* is ineffective. Yet somehow that doesn't prevent us from getting sucked into the well-worn perfection-chasing path.

You know it all too well, be sure to buy your groceries at the farmers' market, organic, of course, and buy only humanely raised, pasture-fed meat. Wait, no, that's not right; only buy food grown within a hundred miles of your home—and just eat plants, because everyone knows meat will kill you. Definitely bring your reusable bags, but wait, scratch that; reusable bags breed harmful bacteria, so that's out too. So maybe just carry everything in your arms? Grab a coffee with coconut oil before you go—no, no, no, coconut oil causes heart attacks. On the way out the door be sure to apply that 100 percent clean, all-natural sunscreen to protect you from damaging UV rays. *Do not forget the sunscreen!* Oh, hold on there, getting vitamin D is actually super-important, so go ahead and skip it. And be sure to rush back, because you need to get your 60 minutes of cardio, every single day. Except, wait; didn't you just read that working out too hard is somehow bad? Maybe you need to study to become a yoga expert instead. Now, where is that ad you just saw for a yoga certification course?

You get the idea; perfectionism is so infused into our daily lives that it almost seems normal. Forget about the fact that the majority of the unrealistic ideals we seek often conflict with one another, and, oh yeah, that part about them being *impossible*? It's a no-win situation. Bottom line, perfectionist thought patterns lead us to believe that the feelings of guilt and of constantly falling short are inevitable. Just a part of life. Mom guilt? Of course. Guilt-related food? Always. Guilt about not getting enough done? For sure.

JANUARY SYNDROME

I've found that perfectionist thought patterns can also pop up when we try something new or try to make changes in our lives. Take January, for example. By now, we all know the drill. New year, new you! Start strong, go all-in, and change everything. But then the reality of life sets in and, after a couple weeks, we end up a little off track. And after a month or so? Well, then we end up completely off track. I call this phenomenon January Syndrome, something I've come to understand well from running a health and wellness website. Although it took me a couple of years to realize exactly *how* important January is in the wellness industry, it did not take long for me to see how perfectionist thinking was the root of the problem. Don't get me wrong; I love the idea of a fresh start as much as anyone, and there's nothing wrong with using January as a time to reflect, step back, and examine our habits and routines.

But the reality is that big goals alone are not enough to sustain change. I know this from the research, but also from witnessing New Year's resolutions from the other side. Running my website all these years has given me an insider's glimpse into the data, including the exact number of people who visit my site each month. And after more than six years of analytics, the trend is clear: January rules. It makes sense that people are interested in personal development, habits, mindset, and eating better in the new year. The interesting thing, though, is what happens right around January 13. About two weeks after the first of the year, after that huge spike on January 2, almost like clockwork, there is a slow and steady decline in traffic. The drop-off continues until sometime around the first week of February, when traffic levels off to where it was in the fall. By mid-February, it's like January never happened. The research supports the January Syndrome drop-off as well, especially when it comes to dieting. Studies have shown that more than 90 percent of people who commit to a diet—no matter what kind—end up regaining any weight they have lost within a year or two at most.

That's the problem with January Syndrome; it places all the emphasis on the glamorous start followed by progress without mistakes, leaving us mind-blind to the realities of life. And with all that focus on *perfect* beginnings, there's no wiggle room or space to handle the inevitable ups and downs of life. The whole premise behind "new year, new you" is that somehow we will suddenly be different. That our life circumstances will have magically changed. But nothing miraculous happens on January 1. That's why the third week drop-off happens. When people feel they aren't living up to unrealistic standards, or when the inevitable mistakes occur, it provides a good enough justification to give up. So we don't need to give up resolutions, or stop trying to focus on eating well, being productive, exercising more, having more positive relationships, or self-love. We just need to know that first we have to ditch the perfection filter in order to find well-being and success along the way. That's the amazing, completely game-changing thing. Because you can absolutely move past this.

Perfectionism Sounds Like . . .

"I can't start until I know exactly how to do it."

"I'll start when I have all the pieces of the puzzle."

"I need to get it all done today: my morning routine, work, eating healthfully, exercising, spending quality time with my partner, being mindful, volunteering, and getting enough sleep."

"I was so busy today, and yet I accomplished nothing."

"If I can't do this the right way, I'm not doing it at all."

The Striving Mindset and perfectionist thought patterns do not have to define you. You can flip the script and take a different path that goes beyond the impossible quest for perfect, and toward something lasting and real. But before we get there, let's take a look at the second part of the Striving Mindset, all-or-nothing thinking.

ALL-OR-NOTHING THINKING

Ah, all-or-nothing thinking. There's just something so seductive about it; right? Go big or go home. My way or the highway. If it isn't a heck yes, it's an *eff* no. This way of thinking is at the core of so many marketing messages that it seems we simply love a good all-or-nothing solution. But here's the problem. This way of thinking frames every choice, every option, and every decision as purely black or white. Two options, two extremes. All-in, or all-out. With nothing in between.

I know it well, as I used to be the poster girl for this on-the-wagon-off-the-wagon approach. I hate to admit it, but I was particularly addicted to all-or-nothing thought patterns when it came to eating. Truthfully, I used to frequently commit to giving up everything I thought I should, *all at once*. "I'm off sugar forever," I'd swear, "and I'm *definitely* giving up all alcohol and, of course, carbs too. Look at me, living this carb-free, sugar-free life!" I'd think, "I've totally got this." And sure, everything would be fine for a while, as I taught myself to deprive my way through temptations and distractions, believing that going all-in was the only way to get results.

Eventually and inevitably, though, the extremes caught up with me, and I'd give up, going all-in instead on everything I'd been restricting. Sometimes I'd cycle between these extremes quickly, each episode lasting just a few days or weeks, while at other times, I'd be able to extend the deprivation cycle for months. Regardless of the time frame, I'd inevitably end up back in the same place. From all-in to all-out, I'd wind up feeling like a giant, hopeless failure in the process. And, boy, would I beat myself up for falling off the wagon. I'd repeat this pattern with exercise—seeking the elusive streak of hour-long workouts—and also at work; after all, if I didn't have a solid hour block to write, what was the point?

FALSE DICHOTOMY

It's actually kind of hard to look back on those years, swinging between extremes. What I realize, now, is that all-or-nothing thinking is a pretty normal part of cognition. Meaning that all-or-nothing thinking, like perfectionist thought patterns, is a normal part of how we are wired—a basic brain design that probably evolved to keep us safe. In fact, our brains are hardwired toward what psychologists call dichotomous thinking, or false dilemma, which means believing that a situation is either/or, when in fact there is at least one other option.

Consider it. If someone in our ancestor group ate a poisonous mushroom and died, it was probably best for the group to rule out *all* mushrooms. No point in taking a risk on the gray area there; right? Dichotomous thinking probably developed to keep us safe. But in our modern lives it seems to have the opposite effect because it makes us think there truly are *only two options*, and then we miss the gray area. And, well, that area is where there's so much more freedom, agency, and choice about how to live.

BURNOUT

If you've ever felt completely burned out, I've got a little secret for ya. Burnout is often a direct result of all-or-nothing thought patterns. It's that part of you that feels like your only option is to go all-in, that can't seem to find a middle ground or an option between extremes. So you go all-in, whether it's a way of eating, exercising, work, or social commitments, all of which might be doable for a while. But then eventually, inevitably, you find yourself exhausted and resentful that you have way too much going on, overwhelmed by everything on your plate, completely exhausted by your day-to-day, or defeated because your needs are yet again at the bottom of the list. This all-in approach sometimes results in burnout, and we may throw in the towel or "fall off the wagon," ending up behind our original starting places.

As I've mentioned, all-or-nothing thinking is a natural reaction in the human brain, but it can also cause a lot of damage when left unchecked. In fact, all-or-nothing thought patterns make people feel worse about themselves and increase anxiety. So if you're feeling bad or particularly anxious, all-or-nothing thinking might be one of the culprits. Add dieting and weight loss into the mix and things get really messy. If you think about it, the hallmark of *any* diet is all-or-nothing thinking. Eat this, not that. Good days and cheat days. Good food and bad food. Given how common all-or-nothing thinking is in dieting, you'd expect there to be some kind of evidence that it works; right? Um, no. All-or-nothing thinking is highly linked in the research with disordered eating and poor body image. Not just that, but it's actually related to weight *gain* in the long term. It will actually land you *behind* the starting line. It's an empty promise, a solution that never works long term.

But wait, you might be thinking, what about those people who achieve greatness through an all-or-nothing approach? Aren't there plenty of examples of athletes and leaders who go all-in, who sacrifice everything, and who accomplish the highest levels of achievement and accomplishment? Yes, it's true. But that's exactly my point. The all-in approach may be one way to achieve success, but it also often requires almost superhuman levels of sacrifice, producing significant negative mental and physical side effects along the way. I don't know about you, but I don't want to sacrifice everything. I don't want to burn out, or feel crushed by anxiety. In truth, I want a life where success doesn't always require such extremes.

All-or-Nothing Thinking Sounds Like . . .

"That weekend pizza-and-wine binge means I'm off the wagon. Might as well have pizza again tonight and skip breakfast and lunch tomorrow to make up for it."

"I don't have time for an hour-long workout, but 10 minutes doesn't really count. Someday maybe I'll find time to work out."

"I'm so burned out on social media. I'm going to delete all my apps and be fully present in my life all the time!"

"I really don't like my job but I can't afford to quit, so I guess I'll just stay and be miserable."

"I've been drinking way too much diet soda lately—only herbal tea for me from here on out."

So, are you doomed to repeat the all-or-nothing cycle and get the same ineffective results? Absolutely not. The good news is that, just like with perfectionism, all-or-nothing thought patterns can be shifted. You have the power to embrace a different way, to get better outcomes and a whole lot more fulfillment along the way. You can exist in the in-between while finding real growth and lasting results. Before we get there, though, we need to cover one more part of the Striving Mindset. Let's talk comparison.

COMPARISON

Hello, comparison. It happens to the best of us; right? Whether it's scrolling social media or simply hanging out with friends. You're going about your business, and then, *bam*, all of a sudden you feel yourself slipping into the comparison trap. Maybe it's catching a glimpse of someone else's seemingly perfect life—his steady stream of photos in exotic travel locations or his brand new car. Maybe it's that mom on Instagram, with her sweet, smiling, perfectly dressed children (*How is she keeping her house so clean when I can't even see my kitchen table under all the clutter?*). Or it's the friend who was recently promoted to his dream job (*How am I still sitting here without a clue of what to do with my career?*). Or it's that couple who seem to have the perfect relationship (*Why does it seem as though they never have an argument, when my partner and I can't stop bickering?*). Regardless of the trigger, we've all been there and know how terrible it feels. The question to ask, then, is if it feels so bad, why do we keep doing it? Social comparison, like perfectionism and all-or-nothing thinking, is a natural part of our brains' function. In fact, our brains are hard-wired to relate information about other people to what we're doing or experiencing. This is one of the main ways humans and other social animals adapt, allowing us to learn from the mistakes of others and not repeat them.

Notice a theme here? Our brains seem to have developed these thought patterns over time as a way to help us, but in our modern world these ways of thinking are doing anything but. And specifically because we seem to be hardwired for comparison, these patterns influence our motivations, how we act, the way we think about ourselves, and ultimately how we feel. There's even research that shows that the brain's reward center lights up not just when you perform well but when you perform *better* than others. In reality, comparison isn't bad in itself, and it can even be useful sometimes. Humans, especially as children, often learn through comparison. And looking around at what other people are doing might inspire you to start something new, to persist when things get hard, or to have hope that good things are possible. Just like perfectionism and all-or-nothing thinking, a little comparison can be a good thing.

The problem is, when left unchecked, it can quickly get out of control. Especially when we have *so many* more opportunities to compare ourselves on a daily basis (hello, social media), the comparison trap can be relentless. And getting sucked into comparison-based thought patterns has serious consequences. Research shows that comparison is a direct contributor to feelings of inadequacy, guilt, shame, and general unhappiness. But you probably already knew that.

TOXIC COMPARISON

I refer to the inadequacy-guilt-shame-unhappiness comparison cycle as *toxic comparison*. It's when comparison goes over the line, from being a source of inspiration to one of devastation. Toxic comparison is so damaging because it keeps you from embracing your own uniqueness; especially if you're trying to start something new. Toxic comparison leads you to believe that you're not doing a good enough job right now, because there's always someone out there doing it better. Toxic comparison is also a big troublemaker when it comes to body image. There's a strong relationship in the research between comparison and body dissatisfaction, and it's highly linked with yo-yo dieting and disordered eating. So basically, comparison is a one-way ticket to feeling like crap about that beautiful body of yours.

I know toxic comparison all too well. Since part of my job includes forward-facing media opportunities, I often get the chance to show up in print and online. This means I'm often *very* visible, right out in the open for everyone to see and scrutinize. It's always been my goal to show up and spread this mission and message; but I'll admit, being so visible is a comparison-fest waiting to happen. In an industry where most wellness leaders are very young and super-fit, it's hard not to compare myself to all those fitness models and clean-eating gurus; and then end up feeling like the way I am is not good enough.

That's the thing about comparison-based thought patterns, there is always someone or something else better, and the way you are does not (and will never) measure up. The bar always rises. On top of that, these patterns cause you to miss the amazingness that makes you uniquely *you*. Think about it. If I were to spend all my time comparing myself to others in the industry, it would stop me in my tracks. I'd shrink down, trying to make myself small, and I'd stop showing up. That's the thing about comparison. It tricks you into thinking you're not good enough as you are; it keeps you playing small and feeling completely miserable too.

Comparison Sounds Like . . .

"She is so much more [stronger, younger, thinner, richer] than I am."

"He's accomplished so much, and I'm just here stuck in the same old place."

"I know I should be grateful compared to other people."

"I thought I was doing fine, but look at how much further ahead of me my friend is. I guess I'm not doing that great after all."

"There is absolutely no point starting this new [way of eating, exercise program, mindfulness practice, work project] because I can't do it as well as the people around me."

So what now? Are you stuck in toxic comparison, sentenced to a life of feeling as though your worth is measured only in reference to someone else's? Of course not. Just like the other two parts of the Striving Mindset, understanding comparison isn't about labeling you, or making you feel bad about the way you think, or assigning shame and blame. Not at all. Pulling back the curtain on comparison-based thinking is simply about knowing that these thought patterns are normal—the way the brain is naturally wired—and, more important, knowing that there are other, better options.

FLIP THE SCRIPT

As you've read, mindset matters when it comes to getting the results you're after. And, as you now know, our brains seem to be naturally inclined toward the Striving Mindset patterns of perfectionism, all-or-nothing thinking, and comparison. The Striving Mindset seems to have developed for a reason; it probably helped us to adapt, stay alive, and thrive over generations.

However, as we now live in a world where avoiding mistakes at all costs and life-and-death choices of friend or foe are not as much a part of the daily struggle for survival, it's time to make some changes. Because striving is not the end of the story. And now that you understand exactly what's happening—and why—you can completely shift the way you think. You can change your brain, which will change your actions, which will change your results, which will absolutely change your life. It's time to move. It's time to grow. It's time to flip the script—from striving and stuck to focused and free.

It's time to feel good.

The Marketing Machine

As we discuss the Striving Mindset, it's probably become obvious just how often you're bombarded with marketing messages that make the mindset worse. When these messages layer on top of our natural brain tendencies toward striving, well, let's just say they make us feel . . . not great. Of course, there are plenty of examples of marketing campaigns that don't try to capitalize on our propensity for perfectionism, all-or-nothing, and comparison. But despite these bright spots, there's still a dark side.

You know what I'm talking about. Those exorbitantly expensive magic powders that tout unlimited energy and improved consciousness, or those before-and-after shots portraying the sought-after flat tummy or ripped physique. The message is clear: You're not good enough the way you are, so try for perfect, go all-in, and make sure you do it exactly like this ideal version that we're offering. Bottom line, our brains are naturally predisposed toward the Striving Mindset, and marketing messages are amplifying the effect. No wonder I spent so many years struggling and feeling bad. No wonder I felt like no matter how hard I tried, I was going nowhere. No wonder it felt like nothing was ever good enough.

THREE

The Feel Good Mindset

Getting clear on the Striving Mindset—perfectionism, all-or-nothing thinking, and comparison—represents a fundamental shift in my own story and experience, as it allowed me to see how flawed many of our commonly held assumptions related to health and happiness are, and therefore, better understand the real reason I'd felt stuck and stressed for so many years. Being able to see this mindset in my own life made it clear why my approach wasn't working.

For the first time in a long time, I felt there was something I could do to move the needle, to make a change, to find a true sense of ease and peace. The only problem was that the sense of relief that came from revealing the Striving Mindset was temporary, because as soon as I understood what was going on, I wanted a way out. I knew there had to be a way to intentionally retrain my brain to counteract the Striving Mindset, to get improved lasting results *and* to actually enjoy the process along the way. So once more, I dug in deep to the research, pulling from positive, behavioral, and cognitive psychology; decision theory; human development; neuroscience; and mindfulness teachings. Taken together, I was able to create an antidote to the Striving Mindset: The Feel Good Mindset.

The Feel Good Mindset is a way of thinking that not only counteracts the Striving Mindset but also is completely actionable; it's a set of thinking skills that can be learned. This means it's not a trait with which you're born, or a personality type that you're stuck in, but, instead, it's a way of thinking that can be learned through practice. So no matter who you are, what your background, or the challenges you've faced, it's available to you. With commitment and consistency, practice and process, you can learn to change your brain. Figuring out the Feel Good Mindset represented a real breakthrough in my story, but the breakthrough paled in comparison to the transformation that occurred when I started putting the new mindset into practice in my own life. All of a sudden, I wasn't trying so hard; I was able to put effort and energy into the things that mattered and to let go of the things that didn't. Without the striving stronghold, I didn't constantly feel guilty or beat myself up about small things. I felt grounded in a foundation of resiliency, and I was able to start living in alignment with my motto: *Gentle is the new perfect.*

By training my brain to use the Feel Good Mindset, I also felt a sense of permission to let my life be real, with all the inherent ups and downs, and to quickly recover when things got off track. My days became so much simpler, too, because I had a clear sense of where to spend my time and energy. No longer operating from a place of scarcity and striving, I was able to celebrate my choices instead of comparing myself to others. I also found that my productivity dramatically increased, as I was no longer procrastinating or scattering my focus and attention across a million actions that didn't matter. For the first time, I understood that wellness need not require restriction, sacrifice, or deprivation and that, instead, joy could be a part of the daily routine. I began getting results *and* enjoying the process along the way. I felt an overall sense of lightness and ease, all while moving forward on the path toward change. This is the power of rewiring your brain. This is the power of the Feel Good Mindset.

This is what I want for you. To shift, to rewire, to feel good. To let go of striving and find a whole new way to wellness. To let it be simple, gentle, and completely sustainable. To create a core of inner resilience so you can handle whatever life throws at you. And to take on life without perfectionism, all-or-nothing thinking, and comparison dragging you down. The Feel Good Mindset is waiting. Let's get started.

WHAT IS THE FEEL GOOD MINDSET?

The Feel Good Mindset is a powerful shift in thinking that will take you from stuck and striving to focused and free. With practice, you'll begin to rewire your brain, which will shift your actions and ultimately change your results.

feel good mindset

SELF-COMPASSION

POWER MIDDLE

GRATITUDE

The Feel Good Mindset is composed of three parts and each part is specifically designed to serve as an antidote to its Striving Mindset counterpart. That is, self-compassion counteracts perfectionism, Power Middle counteracts all-or-nothing, and gratitude counteracts comparison. This means, for example, that if you know perfectionism is a challenge for you, learning self-compassion is going to be life changing.

That said, there's plenty of crossover among the three parts of the Feel Good Mindset, so there's no need to get too wrapped up in the details of matching up everything. The mindset is designed so that focusing on one area of your life will improve the others, and vice versa.

*from striving
to feel good*

PERFECTIONISM ⟶ SELF-COMPASSION

ALL-OR-NOTHING ⟶ POWER MIDDLE

COMPARISON ⟶ GRATITUDE

HOW TO SHIFT MINDSET: THE 4 P'S

I've developed a simple framework to make an easier process of shifting one's mindset. I call it the 4 P's: Pay attention, Pause, Practice, and Patience. Here's how it works.

1   **Pay Attention**
    The first step in shifting mindset is paying purposeful attention to your thought patterns, or the ways in which you're currently thinking. I call this practice micro-mindfulness, taking short moments throughout the day to pay attention to your thoughts.

    The goal is to become aware of your thought patterns—noticing when they come up, and in what context. This simple power of noticing is the first step in sparking mindset shifts. We're going for awareness without judgment here, so try not to use this as an opportunity to beat yourself up; okay? Remember, this isn't about perfect thinking; it's just about nonjudgmental awareness.

2 Pause

The next step in shifting mindset is pause. This involves designating a set amount of time each day to work on mindset. The amount of time need not be long, so starting with 5 minutes is just fine. You'll likely have better success if you assign a time of day for the pause, be it first thing in the morning, in the afternoon, or before bed.

3 Practice

Practice is the next step in shifting mindset, so I've designed daily Mindset Practices for self-compassion, Power Middle, and gratitude to allow you to actively engage in this way of thinking. The practices are designed to fit into your daily life, and I recommend selecting just one to focus on at first. Use your pause time, and consider writing down your practice. I've found that writing serves as a sort of accountability, and there's something about getting the thoughts out of your head and onto paper that seems to lead to better results.

4 Patience

As you apply the first three P's, the effect of mindset shifts will begin to compound. With time, you'll notice how the shifts in thinking positively impact your experience in the world. Taken together, these small moments will add up to a ripple effect across your life.

These shifts do require patience, though. Keep in mind that it took a long time to set the current connections in your brain, most likely years, and will therefore take time and work to reset. Be assured, though, that with practice and time, your brain *will* change.

Tips for Using the Mindset Practices

- Focus on one practice at a time, perhaps starting with the one that speaks to you the most or that you are most likely to remember to use.

- Decide on both a specific amount of time, and a specific time of day to pause and practice. For example, 5 minutes in the morning.

- At first it might seem odd to practice a new way of thinking, especially out of context, which is how some of the practices are designed. With time, you'll be able to put the new ways of thinking into action as the real situation arises.

- Consider creating a mindset journal to capture your thoughts and your practice. Writing helps.

- As you pause, engage, and start to feel the effects, continue to add practices.

- Come back to each practice as needed. Add, subtract, and customize based on what works best for you.

- In need of more structure? Chapters four and ten provide more guidance on creating a personalized practice plan.

SELF-COMPASSION: MOVING AWAY FROM PERFECTIONISM

Self-compassion is the first part of the Feel Good Mindset, as it is perfectionism's kryptonite. Learning self-compassionate thought patterns will allow you to release unrealistic standards, to meet yourself with kindness, and to know that making mistakes is part of being human. It's a way of thinking that will reframe how you view your life, and how you respond to difficult situations. It's so powerful, in fact, that I often wonder why it's not required learning from the time we're young—because the effects of practicing self-compassion are pretty major.

For example, research shows that self-compassion helps people get through difficult challenges, learn from mistakes, and persist even amid difficult situations. It also shows that self-compassionate individuals aim just as high as those without it, yet those who possess it are more resilient if they don't reach their goals the first time around. What's more, this ability to persist and keep going when things get difficult is highly related to self-compassion.

THE RESISTANCE

When I teach self-compassion in workshops and keynotes, I'm often met with strong resistance. People sometimes come to the false conclusion that practicing self-compassion will make them soft, weak, or apathetic. In addition, they mistakenly think that self-kindness is something that's only for wimps and quitters and that adopting a self-compassionate mindset will inevitably take away their competitive edge. This misconception, which seems to be echoed across many cultures—especially in the West—is one that incorrectly assumes success and drive come from being hard on ourselves. We think self-kindness and -compassion will lead to laziness and apathy. Or we think that the only way to achieve results is to tough it out, to put on a hard outer shell, and to push through.

But nothing could be further from the truth. Sure, being hard on yourself might work in the short term, but studies show that people with a strong sense of self-compassion are far more likely to be successful in the long term than people who aren't. Essentially, rewiring your brain toward self-compassion will help you reach your long-term goals. Remember that powerful sting from making mistakes that stems from perfectionist thinking? Well, that sting becomes far less painful when you learn to show yourself kindness, thus increasing the likelihood that you will persist. Also, self-compassion is strongly linked with optimism, self-efficacy, and personal initiative.

Practicing self-compassion, then, results in thinking that things will work out and increases our confidence to do what it takes to reach our goals, without worrying so much about messing it up. Self-compassion also contributes to resilience, which means learning self-compassion will help you better handle setbacks—both big and small—as well as the daily ups and downs of life. Bottom line, if you want to be more productive, to accomplish more, and to be more successful, learn self-compassion.

I also find that sometimes people are resistant to self-compassion because they think that showing themselves the same kindness that they extend to others is selfish. But instead of encouraging selfishness, research has proven that learning self-compassion allows people to *better* take care of others. Research also shows that practicing self-compassion makes for better caregivers, friends, parents, and partners. So, if you want to better serve others, start with self-compassion. Self-compassion is not lazy, weak, selfish, or self-indulgent. It's the opposite.

THE COMPASSION SHIFT

Although self-compassion has transformed my life, I'll admit it was a concept to which I was initially resistant. As someone who used to be incredibly hard on myself, I was skeptical that self-kindness would be of any help. I rolled my eyes. "Oh, please," I thought, "who has time for this nonsense?" Yet the research so strongly supported the benefits that I eventually gave in and began practicing. Pretty quickly I noticed I had more stamina throughout the day, as I wasn't wasting so much mental energy beating myself up about making mistakes. I also noticed that I handled setbacks better than ever, and I had more patience for my family and those around me because I was starting from a place of gentleness with my own shortcomings. I was also able to start, and more important, finish many projects that perfectionist procrastination had once stopped me from making progress on.

Self-compassion has also been a healing balm to my inner bully, one that I didn't even know existed until I started working to change my mindset. As I learned self-compassion, I began to feel a fundamental shift. Small moments of compassion wedged themselves between the internal battle and began to blur the bullying. I stopped trying to meet every unrealistic standard and started to allow myself to be here, as I am, right now. And here's the kicker. Learning self-compassion hasn't made me give up or quit. Actually, this gentle approach has made me stronger, more resilient, and more successful than I ever thought possible. Self-compassion also led to a lot more self-trust, and I couldn't be happier about the transformation.

Practicing self-compassion doesn't mean that every single perfectionist thought pattern disappears entirely. Even as I sit here typing these words, I am aware of the perfectionist thought patterns "This really isn't very good" and "You can do so much better." The difference now, though, is the way I respond. Instead of allowing the thought patterns to derail me, I'm aware of them and I can practice the self-compassionate alternative, which offers the gentle encouragement to keep showing up and continuing to improve. Since I'm not wasting time beating myself up, I'm able to sit through the discomfort when things are imperfect. This book you're holding in your hands? It is the direct result of self-compassion. Of course, your specific perfectionist thought patterns will sound different from mine. Maybe you've never struggled with an inner bully; perhaps unrealistic standards pop up more in relation to your work ethic, your parenting, your athletic ability, or your relationships. Regardless of the trigger, perfectionism is generally easy to identify once you know what to look for because it takes the tone of an inner critic, chastising you for not living up to impossible standards or for not being enough.

At its core, self-compassion is about meeting yourself with kindness and knowing that, as a human, you're bound to make mistakes. It also means knowing that we're all in this together, as self-compassion researcher Dr. Kristin Neff says. Self-compassion is about embracing our common humanity, knowing that we're doing okay just as we are, as perfectly imperfect human beings. Self-compassion is waiting for you. All you have to do is take the first step.

SELF-COMPASSION MINDSET PRACTICES

Because self-compassion requires practicing a different way of thinking, the Self-Compassion Mindset Practices are designed to give you actionable strategies to create this mindset shift.

I recommend picking one practice to start with and then adding others when the first practice starts to become automatic. Know that it's okay if at first the practices feel awkward, uncomfortable, or even silly. If self-compassion is new to you, it will likely feel strange. That's okay. Do it anyway. Practice, and with time, it will become second nature.

PRACTICE: SELF-COMPASSION SCHEDULE

WHAT: Scheduling self-compassion moments into your day.

WHEN: Twice a day. Set an alarm on your phone if you need a reminder.

HOW: Treat yourself to a tiny act of self-kindness by finding a quiet spot to sit and breathe, or taking a short walk. These acts need not be grand or over the top. The point is to start learning to prioritize self-kindness, even if in the smallest of ways.

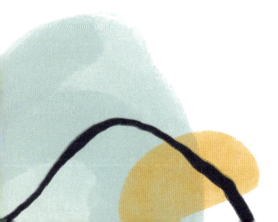

PRACTICE: 5-MINUTE MORNING

WHAT: 5-minute self-compassion morning practice.

WHEN: Set aside 5 minutes in the morning for this practice. It can be longer, but if you struggle to find time for yourself, start with just 5 minutes. If morning isn't an option, set aside time in the afternoon or evening.

HOW: Put away your phone or other possible distractions and use the time to do something kind for yourself. This might include reading, journaling, slowly sipping a cup of tea or coffee, or simply breathing deeply. Use this time to remind yourself that you are worthy of compassion and kindness.

PRACTICE: COMPASSIONATE REFRAME

WHAT: Reframe your internal dialogue to a conversation you would have with a loved one; for example, a child, a partner, a best friend, or even a pet.

WHEN: After making a mistake or when you're being particularly hard on yourself.

HOW: Think about a time when you made a mistake that bothered you. What would you say to your child or a dear friend who made that same mistake? Now repeat those words to yourself, either silently or out loud. Repeat as often as needed.

POWER MIDDLE: MOVING AWAY FROM ALL-OR-NOTHING THINKING

The Power Middle is the antidote to all-or-nothing thinking, as it reframes black-and-white thinking into a multitude of possibilities. It's a way of thinking that allows for gray area, space to explore multiple options, and to experiment with options in between extremes. The Power Middle will allow you to be more flexible in your thinking, and thereby more resilient in your life.

THE POWER OF FLEXIBLE

One aspect of Power Middle thinking is the ability to use a flexible thinking style. This involves allowing for options between extremes and an awareness of the abundance of choices that exist beyond the binary yes/no, in/out, friend/foe. Research shows that people with a flexible thinking style have an easier time dealing with setbacks because they are able to see more alternatives that will allow them to move toward their goals. They also feel better in life because they experience more agency, and thus, more ways to get where they want to go. Researchers have also found that people with flexible thinking are better at handling and performing difficult tasks than those without it. For example, practicing a flexible thinking style allows you to reframe the idea that only extremes count to one in which *everything* counts, be it taking a 5-minute walk, adding a vegetable to your plate, or sitting down to do focused work for a short period of time.

Flexible thinking is also one of the best predictors of avoiding weight gain and having a healthy body weight. Researchers think this is because people who are more flexible in their thinking deprive themselves less and are less rigid about all-or-nothing food rules, achieving better results in the long term. Basically, flexible thinking leads to flexible behavior and the ability to make the most of a situation, regardless of the barriers or obstacles.

THE CIRCLE CYCLE

Another part of Power Middle thinking is the ability to think about time and energy more in terms of circles and cycles than in lines and boxes. This is somewhat of a departure from traditional Western thinking, which often frames them as linear and finite. One need not look far to find such circular progression repeated across the natural world as well. Seasons exist in cycles, each transitioning into another; spring to summer, summer to fall, fall to winter, and winter to spring. What's more, these cycles often occur without clear delineation or stop and start.

Take, for example, physical growth, as measured by height. Thinking about growth linearly causes us to assume that a person's growth can be tracked in a straight line, increasing at the same rate over time. But if you've ever witnessed a child grow, you know that's not how it works. Watching my daughter Elle grow, I've noticed her growth most often occurs in "seasons." Month after month, we'll measure no growth and then, *bam*, seemingly out of nowhere, she'll grow an inch. I would never expect her to grow in equal increments, weekly, yet that's often what we expect from ourselves when it comes to growth toward goals. Similarly, linear thinking often takes the form of thinking in opposites or along a continuum. But when you take the continuum line and bend the ends, that line becomes a circle, which allows for a fuller picture of the abundant options and choices available. Thinking in terms of cycles and circles allows for seasons of effort *and* growth, rest *and* recovery, the natural ebb and flow of life.

Like self-compassion, the Power Middle has both improved the progress I'm able to make toward goals and enabled me to feel good along the way. When I really started to understand that I had the power to find my own way, instead of feeling stuck choosing between two extremes, it opened up so many more options, and allowed me to follow my own path instead of feeling forced into someone else's prescriptive program. Once I started to embrace the Power Middle, I was surprised by just how often all-or-nothing thinking came up in my day-to-day life. I'd catch myself feeling stuck between two options, or struggling with the "this doesn't count" lie. But in noticing all-or-nothing thinking, and practicing Power Middle thought patterns, I was able to give myself permission to count everything, and to once and for all ditch the on-again, off-again wagon mentality. The "I've already ruined it; I might as well start over Monday," or "I had pizza for breakfast, so now I should skip lunch," or "I skipped a few workouts, so I might as well park it on the couch and quit the whole dang thing" approach became a piece of the past because flexible thinking allowed me to know there are always options in between. And instead of seeing growth as a straight, equal line, I could instead see it simply as a series of days, with each offering new opportunities to make choices.

Each day, a new day; each moment, a new moment.

I was actually able to use the Power Middle when I struggled with a cold that just wouldn't quit—nothing serious, just not feeling my best. Resisting the urge to push through (hey, I told you I take self-compassion seriously these days!), I took the week off from exercise, allowing myself time to rest and recover. But you know that in-between-sick-and-well place, where you have to decide if you're going to dive back into your routine full force or whether you're going to take more days to rest? That's exactly where I was. It seemed as if there were only two options: skip another day or dive right back in.

There was, of course, a third option, the place where the Power Middle comes into play. I decided I felt well enough to return to one of my favorite exercise classes, but I made a conscious decision to go back at half speed. This meant that when the instructor told the class to go hard, I maintained at a middle gear. And when she told us to sprint, I kept a steady pace. To be honest, finding a middle ground, especially when the rest of the group is doing something different, can be a little tricky. A big part of me wanted to go all-in, ignore my healing body and just go for it. But by using the Power Middle, I was able to have the best of both worlds. I used flexible thinking about the situation and embraced the season of recovery I was in, knowing that I would be able to circle back to full-effort mode in time. By using this way of thinking,

I was able to resume consistency with my workout routine while also allowing my body time to heal.

That's the thing. Both flexible thinking and thinking in terms of cycles lead to more consistency, rather than less. Remember, consistency doesn't mean doing everything all at once. It means committing to the process and finding consistency in small steps over time.

THE TWO OUT OF THREE RULE

The Two Out of Three Rule is a powerful part of the Power Middle; it will allow you to better embrace a long-term view of success and build a sustainable routine, particularly when you need some equanimity, or sense of stability and calm amid the chaos of life. Apply the Two Out of Three Rule any time you feel you've slipped up or made a mistake or misstep.

Say that your goal is to work out every day this week. But then you miss a day. Applying the Two Out of Three Rule, your goal would be to work out the next two days. Thereby a single missed day becomes less important, and it is less likely to cause you to give in to the all-or-nothing urge. This rule replaces the every-single-day ethos with the simple idea that success is about radical consistency.

Do it more days than you don't.

Show up. Do what you can. Fall down. Get back up. That's what the Two Out of Three Rule is all about. Fair warning, though, this strategy might feel a little uncomfortable at first. I mean, let's take a moment to acknowledge just how totally counter this strategy is to the marketing messages and external expectations you may have internalized over the years. If you were an A student, a high-achiever, or excelled in some other area of life, this can be a tough pill to swallow. I mean, who wants to do something only two out of three times? That's only 65 percent, a C+ at best. So if the idea of two out of three is pushing you out of your comfort zone a little, know those feelings are normal. And, hey, if that never-miss-a-day approach is working for you right now, keep doing what works. If you feel really confident in how you handle setbacks, if life never throws you off your game, if you effortlessly adjust during times of challenge and transition, then this strategy probably isn't for you.

But if you feel what you're doing right now is *not* working, if you find yourself at times feeling on-again/off-again, or struggling to adjust during big life changes, then the Two Out of Three Rule is a great strategy for you. To be honest, it's a strategy that took me some time to adjust to, as well. Trust me, I want nothing more than to work out every single day, to eat beautiful real food 100 percent of the time, to practice mindfulness, to get enough sleep, to get all my work done, to spend quality time with friends and family. I've come to realize, especially since having a family, that I will never have a normal week. Never. Something *always* comes up. Always. This lack of predictability used to drive me nuts. I yearned for the time in my life when I could fit it all in. Since adopting the Two Out of Three Rule, I no longer crave a different life. I'm able to roll with the punches, accepting the unexpected each week, adapting, reworking, and returning to the habits that serve me. To have this simple reframe at my fingertips whenever I'm feeling overwhelmed by fitting it all in, or guilty for slipping up, has changed my life. I think it can do the same for yours too.

Since the Two Out of Three Rule can be applied to just about any situation, let's take a look at some real-life examples. Say your goal is to eat healthful meals every day this week. Then you end up splurging on a night out with friends. You wake up the next day feeling bloated and disappointed that you didn't stick to your original plan. Putting the Two Out of Three Rule into action, you would just focus on the next two meals. You would see breakfast as an opportunity to eat well and hydrate, and lunch as a chance to nourish and restore. The Two Out of Three Rule allows you to stop using past experiences as an excuse and instead helps you focus on the very best choice right in this moment and then move forward. As another example, you miss a workout. Applying the Two Out of Three Rule allows you to focus on the next two workouts. Or if you drop the ball on your mindfulness habit today, focus on getting right back to it tomorrow. Bottom line? When your definition of success changes from getting it right *all the time* to doing what you can *most of the time*, your odds of being consistent go way, way up.

And when your odds for consistency increase, you're able to sustain healthful behaviors long term. Beyond individual opportunities within a particular day (e.g., breakfast, lunch, and dinner), you can also apply the Two Out of Three Rule to entire days and weeks. So if you have a fully "off" day—maybe you're sick, traveling, or taking care of some other responsibility—use the Two Out of Three Rule to focus on the next two days, filling them with nourishment and getting back to basics with your healthful habits. Similarly, if you miss an entire week, focus on the next two weeks. No wasted time and energy feeling guilty or behind. Just forward progress, one day at a time. The rule saves me regularly as a working parent, as I've realized that on most days I can accomplish two things, but often not three. When I really leaned into this realization, when I fully embraced it, everything changed. Most days this means that I can eat well and get my work done, but most likely not get to the gym. With this in mind, I've found ways to slip bite-size pieces of movement into my day, from a quick walk during lunch to firing up a short online workout in the evening. Capitalizing on the two things I *can* do has allowed me to be consistent in my approach to wellness. In truth, the Two Out of Three Rule has saved my sanity. I hope it will help save yours too.

When the Power Middle and Two Out of Three Rule are taken together, a dynamic mindset shift occurs that will allow you to redefine success, use flexible thinking, embrace the phase you're in, and set your own pace in finding radical consistency. Showing up more days than not. That's what the Power Middle is all about.

POWER MIDDLE MINDSET PRACTICES

As with self-compassion, learning Power Middle thought patterns requires a different way of thinking. The Power Middle Mindset Practices are designed to give you actionable strategies to begin creating that mindset shift.

Start with one practice, as you did with self-compassion, adding another when the first practice starts to feel automatic. Again, if at first these practices feel awkward, uncomfortable, or even silly, that's okay. Do it anyway. Practice, and with time, it will become second nature.

PRACTICE: 5-MINUTE RULE

WHAT: When all-or-nothing thinking makes it seem as if there's not enough time or energy, take 5 minutes of action.

WHEN: Use this practice if you feel overwhelmed starting a task because it seems too daunting, or when you feel as though you don't have the time or energy for a task. The trigger for this practice is any time you say to yourself, "I don't have time," or "I don't have the energy." For example, when you notice yourself saying, "I don't have time to exercise," "I don't have the energy to cook dinner," "I don't have time to meal prep," "I don't have the energy to start this work project."

HOW: When you notice this happening, set a timer for 5 minutes. Do as much as you can in that amount of time, then stop. If you can do more, great. If not, that's fine too. Remind yourself that every minute counts.

PRACTICE: THIRD WAY

WHAT: Use this practice when faced with a situation in which there seems to be only two options.

WHEN: The trigger for this practice is if you notice yourself thinking, "It has to be this or that." For example, "I have to finish this entire project, or just give up on it," or "I have to give up my dreams or quit my job," or "I have to train for a marathon or stop running."

HOW: When you notice this happening, write down the two options on a piece of paper. Ask yourself, "Are these really the only two options? Is there a third way?" Challenge yourself to write down as many alternative options as you can.

PRACTICE: ALWAYS, NEVER, RUINED

WHAT: Use this practice when you're feeling stuck in a situation, unable to move forward.

WHEN: The trigger for this practice is when you notice yourself thinking the words "always," "never," or "ruined." For example, "I *always* give up when things get hard," or "I *never* stick with anything," or "I missed a day this week, so now I've *ruined* it."

HOW: When you notice this happening, try reframing it by asking yourself, "Is this true, or are there other possible options?"

GRATITUDE: MOVING AWAY FROM COMPARISON

My guess is that of all the parts of the Feel Good Mindset, gratitude is likely the one with which you're most familiar. Gratitude has entered our collective consciousness in a major way, and for good reason. There are so many benefits of this way of thinking, and if you've already incorporated some kind of gratitude practice into your life, you know just how effective it can be. One of the major benefits of gratitude is that it provides a way out of toxic comparison, allowing you to better see the big picture and to appreciate the goodness that exists in your life at this moment.

MISUNDERSTANDING GRATITUDE

While gratitude is completely amazing, it's also one of those concepts that seems to be a bit misunderstood. There's a common belief floating around that you can't feel gratitude and anxiety at the same time. While I completely understand the spirit of this idea—gratitude has been shown to reduce feelings of anxiety—you can, of course, feel more than one emotion at the same time.

I think we misunderstand gratitude when we approach it with the Striving Mindset, which causes so many problems. To be clear, practicing gratitude doesn't require that you feel grateful 100 percent of the time. It doesn't require that you never feel sad, down, or disappointed. It doesn't mean ignoring the serious issues and challenges in life. I honestly cringe when I hear someone say, "I know I should be grateful when there are so many people worse off than I am, but. . . ." It's that *should* part that gets me. Because ignoring your feelings or comparing your situation to others is not what gratitude is about. Practicing gratitude is instead about training your brain to see the goodness within the tough, difficult, sometimes draining aspects of everyday life. It's a powerful way to rewire your brain to see the reality or full picture of your situation, instead of *just* focusing on the negative.

Because in truth, seeing the negative is another thing that's hardwired into our brains. It's called negativity bias, a natural instinct to identify threat and danger all around us. That's why practicing gratitude is so valuable and so beneficial. Research has shown that people who practice gratitude go on to experience more joy, hope, and love in life, regardless of their individual circumstances. They also experience fewer negative emotions such as envy, greed, and resentment.

A consistent gratitude practice has also been shown to help lessen depression for people with chronic health problems, and it has been linked with increased feelings of trust and empathy, connection, satisfaction, and commitment in friendships, romantic relationships, and marriages. So, yeah. It's that good.

USING GRATITUDE TO UNDO NEGATIVITY BIAS

Gratitude can be used to counteract negativity bias; another one of those things that probably developed to keep us safe from real danger. Think about it. In ancient times, if you were constantly on the alert, looking for threats, you were more likely to survive. You wouldn't get eaten by the lion because you were vigilantly on the lookout. These days our brains are hyperaware of threats that aren't really dangerous. Negativity bias is the reason that a rude comment you receive on social media stands out far more than the dozens of positive ones. It's the reason you can remember the exact words of criticism you received back in high school, even though you can't remember the names of most of your classmates. And it's the reason that all the things that went wrong during the day pop into your head right before you fall asleep. Negativity bias is also highly related to toxic comparison because it causes you to overfocus on the bad, stressful, or threatening things in daily life, instead of seeing the reality of the situation. That's exactly what makes it so insidious—it gives more weight to the bad things, causing you to miss so much of the good.

But that's where gratitude comes into play. Gratitude neutralizes negativity bias, allowing you to see more of the story beyond immediate threats. Practicing gratitude essentially creates a *positivity bias*, one that allows you to see a fuller picture of your experience—the negative *and* the positive—as well as know that your worth, and value, has nothing to do with anyone else. More accurately, gratitude essentially creates a *reality bias*, one that's grounded in the full spectrum of what is real, both the good and the bad.

SHOULD TO GOOD

Take a moment to think about how often the word "should" comes up in daily conversation. "I *should* work out more," "I *should* get around to organizing my closet," "I *should* start meal prepping," "I *should* be more productive." The thing about "should" is that it often exists as a proxy for comparison, representing a focus on what everyone else is doing, rather than what would be good for you. When "should" pops up in my thinking, I've learned to reframe it in terms of "good," or what would be good for me right now. *Should to Good* is a strategy to use gratitude to focus on your own story, your uniqueness, and what actually works for you. Of course, most of us know, at least on some level, that just because something worked for someone else doesn't mean it will work for us.

But it can be so easy to fall into the one-size-fits-all trap, thinking that if it *does* work for someone else, it *should* work for us. Researchers call this the patient uniformity myth. For example, when it comes to randomized pharmaceutical and therapy clinical trials, "proven effective" only means that the drug or intervention worked for about 50 percent of the people tested. That said, placebos often work on 25 to 33 percent of those tested, so some of the best researched and "proven effective" medicines and treatments will actually work on 15 to 25 percent of those who use them. Now I'm definitely not saying that it's bad to use treatments that have been proven effective. Having a gold standard in medicine is important, and clinical trials are very useful in determining what works best for an aggregate of the population. But the idea that one thing will work for everyone, without taking into account individual life circumstances and other variations? Well, that's just a myth.

THE OWN IT ZONE

Despite all the research on the benefits of gratitude, when I first started practicing I honestly didn't expect much. "How can the simple act of focusing on what I'm grateful for make any real difference?" I asked myself. Once I learned how to shift my thought patterns toward gratitude, I was surprised at just how much it changed my daily experience. Focusing on the bigger picture allowed me to feel a sense of grounded calm. I no longer went to bed each night hyper-focused on a long list of things going wrong in my life. You, too, can abandon the one-size-fits-all approach and use gratitude to take what's available and make small tweaks and adjustments for *you*, creating what is essentially your own customized approach. Once this customization happens, there's no need for comparison because what you've created is right for you alone. One of my favorite ways of using gratitude is to designate Own It Zones.

An Own It Zone is that beautiful place where you ditch the FOMO (fear of missing out) and embrace your own, unique life. Finding your Own It Zone is kind of like creating your personal gratitude-based life recipe. Customize the little things and use gratitude to draw attention to your preferences so you can create spaces, routines, and habits that are built for you. Own It Zones can be created for just about any part of life, from your workouts to the way you eat to relationships. I used my gratitude practice to create an Own It Zone by homing in on the parts of movement that allow me to feel good. For example, while hiking I'm able to tune in to gratitude related to my senses and felt experiences. Hiking becomes my Own It Zone, one that I come back to whenever I get a twinge of jealousy or the urge to compare. Instead of comparing myself, I just smile because I have my Own It Zone, my own thing that works for me.

You can also apply Own It Zones to your style of eating, particularly if the diets or meal plans you've tried haven't worked for you. Starting with gratitude and noticing your preferences, tune in to how your body feels in relation to what you're eating.

The key here is to experiment in your own life, notice gratitude, and, once you've settled on something, really own it. No need to apologize, second guess, or look around at what everyone else is doing. Because when you've figured out what works for you, it becomes effortless to ditch comparison in favor of your beautiful, unique self.

GRATITUDE PRACTICES

As with self-compassion and Power Middle, learning gratitude thought patterns requires a different way of thinking. These Gratitude Practices are designed to give you actionable ways to shift your mindset. Start with one practice at a time, adding another once the first practice starts to feel automatic.

If any of the gratitude rituals feel awkward or forced, that's okay. Practice and, with time, they will become second nature. Remember, too, that gratitude doesn't mean you are always happy or thinking positive thoughts. You can feel grateful and all kinds of other feelings at the same time. It's just about bringing more awareness to the good.

PRACTICE: THREE GRATEFUL THINGS

WHAT: Create a simple gratitude practice to reflect on the things for which you are grateful each day.

WHEN: Pick a time of day, such as first thing in the morning or right before you go to bed at night.

HOW: Every day write down three things for which you're grateful. No need to journal for hours, just a quick, simple list will do. You might want to create a specific gratitude journal for this purpose. If you feel stuck, start with small details. So instead of writing a broad general list, try getting specific; for example, the way morning light hits your comforter, the smell of coffee, the sound of your partner's laugh.

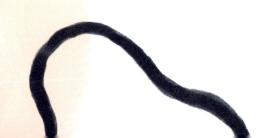

PRACTICE: GRATITUDE FILES

WHAT: Capture small moments of gratitude using the camera on your phone. Then move the images into a specific gratitude file.

WHEN: Daily. Consider setting an alarm on your phone for a certain time of day and then take a photo at that time.

HOW: Challenge yourself to capture at least one photo per day. If you're feeling stuck, look for tiny details. Return to the file whenever you need a little reminder, or a fuller picture, of all the ways gratitude shows up for you on a daily basis.

PRACTICE: STOP, DROP, GRATITUDE

WHAT: A minute of gratitude.

WHEN: Use this practice during specific moments of comparison. For example, when you notice yourself comparing your current situation to someone else's or to another time in your life, or when you're feeling like you're not making progress toward a goal.

HOW: When you notice comparison happening, stop, set a timer for 1 minute, and focus your attention on one thing you're grateful for. If you're stuck, focus on small details—your breath, the feel of the air on your skin, a favorite sound or song, a pleasant smell, etc.

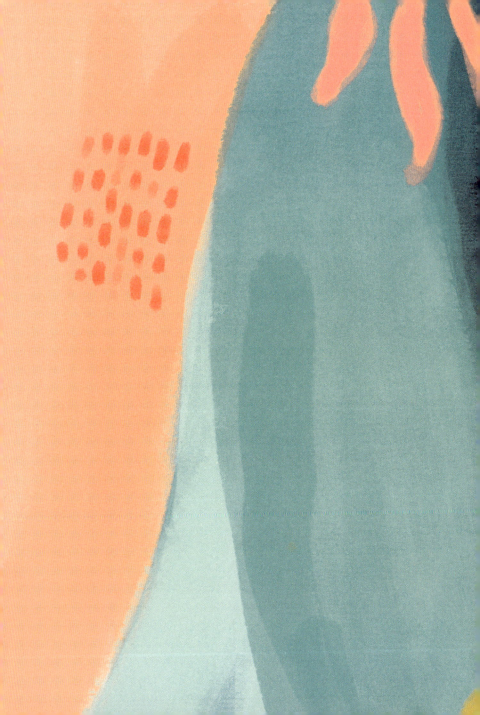

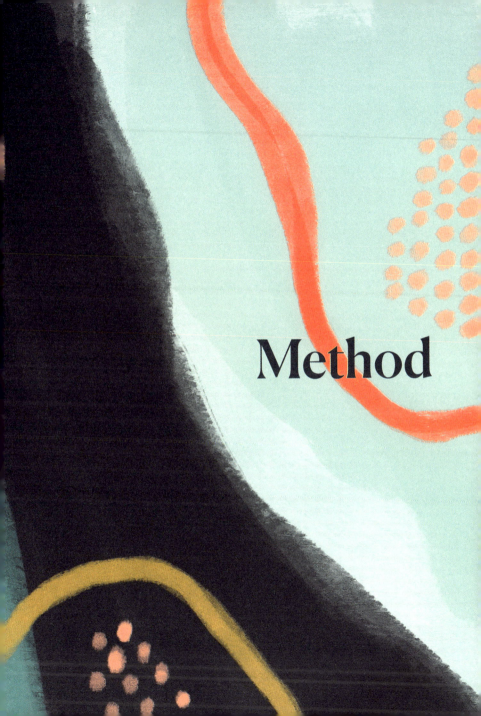

Method

FOUR

The GOOD Method

Well, hey there! So glad you made it. By now you should feel pretty amazing knowing that you have a solid grounding in the Feel Good Mindset, including an arsenal of quick and effective practices to help you shift your mindset for good. In this section, we're going to focus on creating simple systems to help you commit, find consistency, and get the results you're looking for.

A (BETTER) SYSTEM FOR RESULTS

So now maybe you're wondering, What exactly is a system anyway? That's a very good question, as it's often a lack of effective systems that causes things to begin to fall apart in your quest for results. I mean, think about the last time you tried to change something in your life. My guess is that you probably tried to create a new habit or start a new routine or strategy. Perhaps you decided to start working out, or eat better, or become more productive. But after a few days or weeks, you fell into your old ways.

If this sounds familiar, you're not alone—this scattershot approach to change is all too common. The problem is, it simply doesn't work. The reason? There was no system in place to help support the change you were seeking to make. Essentially, a system is an organized method to achieve a result, or a set of things working together in an inter-connected network to accomplish a goal. It's this connection of parts working together toward an outcome that makes systems so effective.

This is the reason that focusing on habits or strategies absent other factors rarely works. So much wasted effort, with so little payoff at the end. That's why I've created a system that takes into account the major players when it comes to change and organizes them together to get the results you desire. It's the synergy of habits, strategies, and mindset working together that's so powerful. Let's take a look at each part.

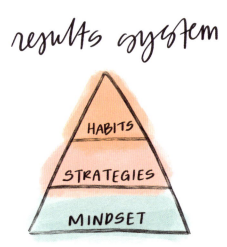

HABITS: WHAT

Habits are the specific actions you take—your tasks and routines. Remember when I told you that habits make up 45 percent of your daily behavior? Think of them as the "what," or what you do every day.

STRATEGIES: HOW

I like to think of a strategy as a collection of habits working together toward a result. Strategies, then, are the "how," or how you take action.

MINDSET: WHY

As you now know, mindset is the way you think—your specific thought patterns. Within this system, then, think about mindset as the "why," or why you take specific actions.

Taken collectively, you can see why it's the system of all three—habits, strategies, and mindset—that has the potential to move the needle in a very big way. Trying to adopt a strategy without having the mindset in place is a scattershot approach; without supporting thought patterns, you're bound to repeat the same old actions, ending up with the same results. Similarly, trying to add new habits without strategy means the habits have nothing to stick to. And mindset without strategy and habit ignores that "how" and "what" of real life. That's why in this section we'll put it altogether; using the Feel Good Mindset and the GOOD Method to get you the results you're after.

HOW THE GOOD METHOD WORKS

The GOOD Method is a set of four science-based, life-tested habits and strategies designed to work with the Feel Good Mindset. Together they create a system to support the results you want in life; to help you prioritize what matters, to make better decisions, and to automate better habits. And while plenty has been written about prioritization, habit, and decision making, the goal of this system is different. It's designed to support a purposeful, feel-good life. Working synergistically, the Feel Good Mindset and the GOOD Method create a system of small shifts that amplify each other, creating long-term, sustainable results.

good method

G OAL FLIP

O UTLAST

O PTIMIZE TO SATISFICE

D ECISION DIET

GOAL FLIP

Goal Flip is a strategy to support the prioritization and automation of specific habits that get results.

OUTLAST

Outlast is a strategy to support the prioritization and automation of specific habits to help you persist and be consistent long term.

OPTIMIZE TO SATISFICE

Optimize to Satisfice, or pursuit of a satisfactory outcome, is a strategy to support better decision making through the identification of trade-offs.

DECISION DIET

Decision Diet is a strategy to support better decision making by reducing decision fatigue.

MAKING THE MOST OF THE METHOD

At a time when much wellness advice takes the form of prescriptive diets, detailed workouts, and predetermined plans, the GOOD Method is specifically designed to offer flexibility and customizability for your life. It's not another fad diet, a gimmicky workout, or a get-happy-quick scheme. Instead, it's a solid framework to help you make small shifts for big change. It allows you to figure out what actually works for you, in your life, and with your own set of preferences, circumstances, and values.

That said, if you're used to following rigid programs, doing the work to customize a system might feel uncomfortable at first. Believe me, I know that it can be tempting to want someone to give you an exact plan. I understand, too, that trying something new, learning to listen to your life, and trusting yourself can be challenging. But hear me out. This is going to be worth it because prescriptive programs simply do not work over time. If you've already tried quick fixes that haven't worked for long, I hope you'll give this alternative system a try. So as we dive in to this next section, I invite you to do the following.

Allow yourself room to be a beginner.

Treat this like an experiment, to create feedback loops in your life about what works, and what doesn't.

Make small changes that will enable major shifts.

Think of these small changes connecting to something bigger—a constellation of actions that together will lead to health, happiness, and feeling good.

Start where you are.

Take what you need; leave what you don't.

You are absolutely capable. And that small voice in your head that whispers what's best? It's about to get a whole lot louder. Are you ready? Let's start by figuring out *your* feel good.

MAKE IT HAPPEN EXERCISES

I begin each episode of the Feel Good Effect podcast by encouraging listeners to "make it happen." Making it happen means taking action, because while it's great to learn new things, it's taking action that actually propels you forward. Located at the end of the following chapters in this section, you'll find Make It Happen Exercises, designed to help you put the information you've learned into action. Know that the exercises are meant to complement and amplify one another, so start with one and add on as you go, thereby creating a powerful upward spiral of momentum. You'll also find a game plan to get started as part of the challenge outlined in chapter ten.

Vision

In 2017, I created the Feel Good Effect podcast to answer a simple question: What does it really mean to be healthy? This question arose because as I looked around at the health and wellness industry, the answer didn't seem exactly clear. Did "healthy" mean adaptogenic smoothies? Gurus and meditation retreats? HIIT workouts and spin classes? Or, I wanted to know, was there more, a deeper meaning to the humble word?

Over the years, I've posed this question to more than a hundred guests on the show, all health and wellness visionaries and innovators. After I ask the question, almost inevitably, they pause, sometimes caught off guard or struggling to come up with a succinct response right away. After some reflection, however, most give an answer that sounds a lot like this: "Healthy" means feeling good, in mind, body, and soul.

These answers inevitably reach beyond the specific types of food we eat or the workouts we do. Instead, they get to the core of the question—that healthy is about feeling good. Which, of course, begs the follow-up question: What does it mean to feel good? What I've learned over the years is that there are as many answers to this question as there are people to whom it's posed. And that's the point.

It's your personal definition that matters. When *you* define "feeling good," you can then adopt specific strategies and habits to align with that definition. That's why I created the Feel Good Vision exercise (see page 86), to help you create a specific vision and definition of what feeling good means to you.

MAKE IT HAPPEN EXERCISE: FEEL GOOD VISION

This exercise is a variation on a more traditional values exercise, which I've adapted to allow you to define your unique vision of feeling good. Crafting this specific, personalized vision will allow you to utilize it as a guiding star, something to orient toward, align with, and use as you navigate the remaining chapters in this book and beyond.

1   On a piece of paper, brainstorm a list of ten words representing how you want to feel in life. Feeling stuck? Set a 10-minute time limit and write anything that comes to mind. You may also use the following list as inspiration.

activated	energized	joyful
adventurous	focused	open
calm	free	peaceful
centered	generous	present
clear	grounded	resilient
connected	independent	vibrant
courageous	innovative	

2   Circle the five words that most resonate with you. No need to over-think it; just circle the first five that pop out.

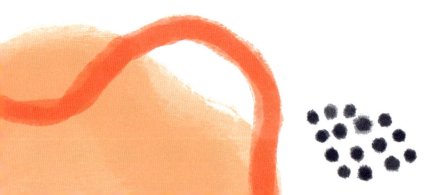

3   Next, on a separate piece of paper, write "feel good" in the middle, drawing a box around the words.

4   Surrounding the box, write the five words you selected, circle each, and draw lines from the box to them.

5   Around each circled word, write all the reasons *why* you want to feel that way, drawing a line from each word to the whys.

6   Now select the three circled words with the most connected whys.

7   These three words represent your Feel Good Vision—your guiding star. Write them down as a reminder. Place them in a visible location. Come back to them often and use them as you navigate the remaining chapters in this book and beyond.

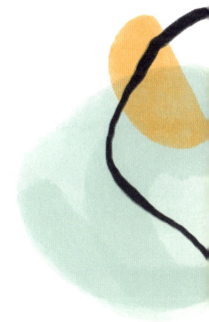

FIVE

Goal Flip

Goal Flip is the first part of the GOOD Method, designed to help you prioritize and automate daily habits to get results. Goal Flipping reframes traditional goal setting by switching your focus to the *process* instead of the *outcome*. It's a more-effective strategy than traditional goal setting because although the commonly held belief seems to be that change comes simply from setting better goals and then trying harder, that's not really how it works.

In fact, research has shown that people who focus on *outcome* goals—things such as losing weight, getting better muscle tone, or becoming more attractive—are less likely to meet their goals than people who set *process* goals—things such as having fun, working out with friends, or meeting new people. Speaking for myself, I know traditional goal setting doesn't work because of my personal history of trying (and failing) to reach outcome-based goals. Believe me, I've tried all the traditional goal-setting strategies, from creating SMART (specific, measurable, attainable, relevant, and timely) goals to downloading fancy apps that track my progress to buying all kinds of planners and journals.

I even signed up for a half marathon, thinking that it would force me to finally start running constantly. Yet in reality, the half-marathon goal was kind of a disaster. Since I wanted to start running more, but didn't know where to begin, I figured setting a goal to run a half marathon would give me the motivation to actually do it. I'll admit that setting such a big goal felt really good. I felt cool telling people about my plans, and I had visions of myself completing the race, running across the finish line, hands in the air, feeling accomplished and victorious. It just felt so great to sign up, and printing out a three-month detailed training plan gave me such a sense of satisfaction. Finally, I had a SMART goal, and I had a plan.

FAILURE STATE

In the weeks following my half-marathon decision, I stuck to the training plan. The only problem was that I *loathed* the training. As in, I legit hated it. I dreaded the long-run days, and my body felt beat up for days after. The only thing keeping me going was the promise of that end goal, the day I'd run victoriously across the finish line. Now think about this; I trained for three months and completed training runs about five days a week. That's a total of sixty days, give or take a few days, training for the goal. Now, consider, it took me just *one day* to run the half marathon. So essentially I spent 1 percent total of my time actually reaching the goal. Which means I spent 99 percent of the time *not* reaching it. No matter how you look at it, that is a lot of time not reaching the goal. I call this failure state, meaning that in pursuit of a goal we spend the majority of the time actively failing to reach it. Now I don't know about you, but I'd rather spend the majority of my time meeting my goals, not the other way around.

Another issue that arises from operating in a failure state is the significant drop-off that typically occurs once the goal is met. It's probably not hard to guess what happened the week after I completed that half marathon. Yeah, I stopped running. I'd met the goal, and hated the day-to-day process of getting there. Sure, I could have trained for another race; but in the end, the short-term endorphin high of reaching the goal simply wasn't enough to sustain the daily habit of running. Andrew, on the other hand, loves running. For him, running the forest trails near our home offers both a fantastic form of exercise and an essential way to relieve stress. Like me, he decided to set a race goal, though his was to run and complete a full marathon. In setting this goal, his intention was to make running a higher priority. Unfortunately, he didn't fully take into account his workload, family responsibilities, and the rigor of his training plan. Ultimately he made it all work; but by the time he ran the race, he felt depleted and, ironically, more stressed than when he'd started. The activity that had once served as a valuable form of stress relief had turned into the source of it.

Now maybe you've never set a goal to run a distance race, but per-haps instead you've set an outcome-based goal of getting 10,000 steps a day or closing all the rings on your fitness tracker every single day. If you've ever set these types of outcome-based goals, you know that at first they can be very motivating. Perhaps the goal inspires you to get up and move, and the activity feedback is informative and helpful. But then perhaps you miss a day. And then maybe two. You forget to wear your tracker and feel as though your workout didn't "count" because your rings remain unclosed. Maybe you got sick or injured, or the 10,000-step goal wasn't quite realistic in the first place. Then—and I'm just guessing here—you decided to *stop wearing the fitness tracker.* Because who wants a pedometer or tracker reminding you that you're failing? There's probably a proverbial fitness-tracker graveyard some-where, littered with tracking devices cast off because of this reason. Or, maybe, hitting your daily goals or closing the rings becomes some-what of an obsession, and what was once a helpful way to track activity devolves into something else entirely. Either way, I'm not saying to ditch running goals altogether, avoid signing up for marathons, or give up your fitness tracker. Not at all. I'm just saying there are additional ways to get results.

DELAY DISCOUNTING

When you set outcome-based goals, a secondary problem can also arise, and that is what it does to your focus. When you set a goal for weeks, months, or years in the future, you automatically start living for the future. Think about that for a second. It's pretty hard to be present, to focus on what's happening right now, when you're con-stantly thinking about what's to come. What's more, setting future goals causes you to lose sight of those day-to-day actions that actually lead to results.

In addition to taking your focus away from what needs to happen today, future goals also can cause you to expend precious mental energy thinking about things that haven't happened yet. More than that, as soon as the goal starts to seem improbable or impossible, the odds of quitting go way up, meaning that the temporary burst of motivation that results from setting the goal evaporates quickly. Psychologists call this delay discounting, meaning that a reward loses value the further off it is in the future.

Here's how delay discounting works. Imagine I offer to give you $100 today or $110 tomorrow. Which would you choose? Studies have shown that people are most likely to choose the $110 option because waiting an extra day is worth the extra $10. But now imagine I offer to give you $100 today or $110 in a month, or a year, or in ten years. Studies have also shown that for the majority, the extra $10 is not worth the cost of waiting for it. Delay discounting means that *things literally lose value the longer we have to wait for them.* Our hardwiring toward immediate gratification means that setting far-off goals offers an initial burst of motivation but, since it's the day-to-day actions that actually get results, that small burst simply isn't enough to sustain us over time.

PROCESS OVER GOAL

If traditional, outcome-based, future-focused goal setting doesn't work long term, what's the alternative? Because, if you're like me, you still want to do great things. You want big results, and you want results that *last*. You're not looking to go one and done, and you don't want to sign up for the race only to quit during the training process, or the day after the race is completed. So I'm not saying to give up on your goals, whether that involves eating better, exercising more, writing a book, starting a podcast, switching careers, or going back to school. Whatever it is you want to do, you can still do it. This isn't about giving up on your dreams. It's the opposite.

Process Over Goal is a strategy that switches focus from the end outcome to the process of what it takes to get there. Recall that people who set process goals reach them faster and more often, and maintain them in the long-term. Research also shows that people who set process goals are also significantly *happier* all along the way. It's by focusing on the process, the day-to-day actions, that gets you lasting, real results, and actually enjoy getting there. It requires a reframe to focus on the day-to-day and the small actions, to stop living for the future, to create change that actually lasts, and to find joy in the process.

FLIP IT UP

Now that you know what Process Over Goal means, let's talk about the tactical strategy of doing it in daily life. I call this technique Goal Flipping. One of my favorite examples is in the coaching strategy of Nick Saban, currently head coach at the University of Alabama and arguably one of the greatest coaches in collegiate football history. Whether or not you're a fan of football, there's no denying that Saban's coaching strategies are effective. At the time of this writing, his record is 237-63-1; as a head coach he's won 237 out of 301 games, meaning an almost 80 percent win record. For context, that level of success in collegiate football is unprecedented. You'd think, then, that one of the most successful coaches of all time must use traditional goal-setting techniques. You'd think that Saban must have his team set SMART goals, visualizing winning national championships and focusing their attention on beating every opponent.

But that is not what he does. Instead, Coach Saban Goal Flips. Admittedly, I'm sure *he* doesn't call it Goal Flipping but, nevertheless, his technique illustrates perfectly the strategy. Saban doesn't talk to his players about winning national championships, or conference titles, or even the next game. He talks about *what's now*. Each day at practice or at game time, he coaches his players to hyper-focus on executing a specific play, or series, or skill, to the best of their abilities. They're not looking at the future or reflecting on the past. They put a constant focus on moving forward by looking at today, one action at a time. And can you guess what happens as a result of this strategy? His team wins. His team wins a lot. They win games. And conference titles. And national championships. Not by looking ahead but by focusing on the process of what's right now. They don't give up on results by ditching outcome-based goals. They use process-based goals to get *better* results.

This is what I want for you too. I want you to win. I just want you to win one day at a time. And I want you to do it with just a little bit of joy. Now, I don't know Nick Saban personally, but I'd be willing to bet that he is not particularly concerned about making the process joyful for his players. I add joy into the Goal Flipping strategy because I know—both from experience and from the research—that making the process enjoyable will allow you to succeed long term. I personally use Goal Flipping any time I want a result. In fact, I used it to write this book. Instead of setting a traditional goal, I Goal Flipped by focusing on the daily process and the actions required to move forward toward the result of a completed book. To get to a completed book, the process is surprisingly simple. It's sitting down and writing words. Not thinking about the book. Not researching for the book. Not talking to people about the book. But sitting down and writing words. Yes, thinking, and researching, and talking can all be part of the process. But the daily action of actually sitting down, in front of the computer, and writing words? That's the process. Not what's *next*. Just what's *now*.

And here's the thing you should know. The process? It's often the thing we most often want to procrastinate and avoid. The hard truth is that setting an outcome-based goal often feels glamorous and exciting. We want to think that setting the goal is the same thing as doing the work, or taking the action, day in and day out. But the magic is *in* the process. There is magic in getting out of a failure state, of living for today instead of for the future, of doing the actual work. Sitting down and writing the words. Focusing on the process, even on the days when you don't feel like it, or when it's messy, imperfect, and incomplete. Especially on those days. Because, spoiler alert: The process often is messy, imperfect, and incomplete. But that's why we have the Feel Good Mindset—self-compassionate, Power Middle, grateful progress. Gentle over perfect, one step at a time.

MINI-MILESTONES AND BIG WINS

It's important to note, too, that Goal Flipping does not mean you have to give up on a sense of progress or growth. Both are essential to health and happiness, so documenting them is a key part of the Goal Flipping strategy. Documenting progress toward a completed book, then, starts by asking a new set of questions. Questions like, "Am I sitting down and writing words?" If yes, that's good; this is the progress in the process. The day I submit the first draft of the manuscript, then, becomes a part of the process to be documented and acknowledged. Similarly, the day the book is published is another part of the process to be documented and celebrated. These all represent big wins, and you better believe I celebrated them. But still. They *are* part of the daily process. Never the end. Always a way forward.

In this process, documenting progress involves establishing what I call Mini-Milestones and Big Wins. Both keep you motivated and infuse joy into the day-to-day and are ways to mark forward progress, allowing you to celebrate the present moment, and to feel a sense of growth along the way.

Mini-Milestones in the process of writing a book might include:

> Writing for three hours a day, for four out of five days this week.

> Completing a full draft of a chapter by the end of next week.

And a Big Win in the process of writing a book might include:

Finishing a draft of an entire section.

Finalizing the cover design.

Turning in the first draft of the manuscript.

Completing the final page proofs.

With Mini-Milestones and Big Wins, you're able to feel a sense of momentum and progress, and you'll be able to pause to enjoy the journey.

REFUSE TO HATE THE PROCESS

Goal Flipping also requires that you intentionally infuse joy into the process. Infusing joy is necessary because there will be many days when the process will not feel sexy, shiny, or exciting. Real results come from work, commitment, consistency, and effectively navigating discomfort and challenge. But that doesn't mean it always has to suck. The idea that you have to suffer for success is just plain wrong. To be clear, infusing joy doesn't mean you have to love every second of the process, or that the act of change, growth, and forward progress will not be uncomfortable and challenging at times. But it doesn't require martyrdom. You can resist. You can *refuse to hate the process*. Because the process is your life.

Infusing joy into the process of book writing for me includes playing my favorite music in the background, writing in a comfy chair with a cozy blanket at hand, having a mug of my favorite coffee (morning) or tea (afternoon) nearby, and diffusing my favorite oils on the bookshelf next to my desk (orange and vanilla, if you're wondering), plus taking stretch- and walk-breaks when my body needs a respite from sitting. Simple, small things to make the day-to-day a little more enjoyable.

Taken altogether, Goal Flipping is a strategy that will allow you to focus on the process, the daily set of actions that move you in the direction toward your desired results. Forward momentum, one day at a time. If it's running, it's lacing up your running shoes and putting in the mileage. If you're writing a book, it's sitting down and writing the words. If you're trying to change the way you eat, it's shopping for, preparing, and eating real food. And it's infusing little joys so you can stick with it in the long term. It's feeling the satisfying soreness that comes from a week of exercise; finding satisfaction from writing the words, even if they aren't good at first; or knowing the gratification of fueling your body with healthful food. Focus on the process, take the daily actions, find the joy, and do it again, and again, and again. Then watch how things begin to change.

MAKE IT HAPPEN EXERCISE: GOAL FLIP

If you're ready to put Goal Flipping into action in your life, use this Make It Happen Exercise for the step-by-step.

START WITH A RESULT

Choose a specific result that you'd like to move toward. Maybe it's changing the way you eat to focus on whole foods, moving your body on a regular basis, or clearing the mental clutter so you feel calmer and more at peace. Perhaps it's building a business or writing a book. Just get clear on the results you're after. Write the result at the top of a piece of paper.

Hint: I recommend referring back to your Feel Good Vision words (see page 86). You might consider selecting one of your words as a result.

REVERSE ENGINEER

Working backward, reverse engineer the result by identifying the specific set of daily actions and habits that will create the result. List them under the result on the same piece of paper.

MINI-MILESTONES + BIG WINS

Establish Mini-Milestones and Big Wins to keep you focused and feeling as though you're making progress. Think about Mini-Milestones as daily to weekly progress markers, and Big Wins as progress you can celebrate and savor along the way. Write lists of both on the same piece of paper.

INFUSE JOY

Check for joy; identify opportunities to infuse pleasure into the process.

Hint: Ask yourself, "How can I feel good while doing it?" "What small joys can I add to make the process more engaging?" Write these on the paper.

You now have a process blueprint for creating big results. Refer back to this piece of paper to maintain focus on the process, and celebrate those Mini-Milestones and Big Wins. Know, too, that the more you practice Goal Flipping using this exercise, the easier it will become. You'll quickly be able to reverse engineer any results, identify the daily process, make progress, and enjoy yourself along the way.

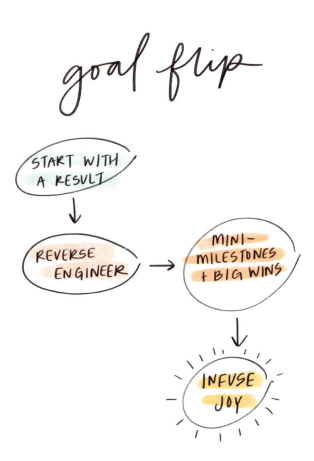

SIX

Outlast

If you're anything like me, you're probably quite familiar with daily to-do lists. To be honest, I used to harbor a bit of a to-do-list obsession. Just so you know, I'm one of those people who will put an item on a list for the simple satisfaction of crossing it off. But over time, I've come to realize that my past approach to list making wasn't really serving me. For years I'd create lists upon lists, always starting with just a few tasks but inevitability adding more, more, and more, until the list became so long and daunting that I'd feel completely overwhelmed, eventually giving up on trying to get any of it done.

In the times when I was able to gather the energy to work through the list, I'd often become paralyzed, unsure of what to prioritize. I thought everything on the list was equally important, that it all mattered, and that it all mattered *a lot*, therefore creating the false sense that prioritization was impossible. What I realize now is that I was operating under the faulty assumption that everything matters equally, which meant that I was wasting time and energy trying to get it *all* done, and therefore unable to prioritize what actually mattered. Operating under this false assumption, I hustled trying to do everything, running in circles trying to keep up and then quitting under the sheer magnitude of it all. But eventually, I learned the truth.

EVERYTHING DOES NOT MATTER EQUALLY

The truth is that everything *does not* matter equally. Seriously, let that sink in. And because everything does not matter equally, there are just a few actions and habits that matter a *whole lot more* than everything else. Here's the deal. Have you ever heard of Vilfredo Pareto? He was an Italian economist in the early 1900s who noticed that 80 percent of results come from 20 percent of actions. This observation is now known as the Pareto principle, or the 80/20 rule. Pareto's principle means that it's a mere 20 percent of effort in any given area of life that actually moves toward results.

Over the past century, the 80/20 rule has been proven in everything from business to technology to relationships. For example, research has shown that light physical activity—things such as standing, walking, doing light housework, or moving your body in a comfortable way without necessarily sweating or even breathing hard—has almost the same health benefits as more intense exercise. Some studies have found that the biggest health benefits—things such as lower risk for cancer, heart disease, and diabetes—don't come as a result of the intensity of exercise but rather from simply spending less time sitting. In other words, doing a workout that is too hard or that you don't like is not only unnecessary but it potentially keeps you from focusing on what really matters—the 20 percent that yields 80 percent of health benefits. Which is actually just getting up and moving in a way that feels good to you.

Other studies related to happiness have shown similar effects. Specifically that of all the ways people spend effort, time, and money in pursuit of happiness, only five variables really seem to make a meaningful difference in well-being, happiness, and life satisfaction: experiencing positive emotions, engaging in work and/or hobbies, having strong relationships with family and friends, feeling a sense of meaning in life, and possessing a sense of accomplishment in working toward goals. That's it—those five things make up the 20 percent that leads to 80 percent of our happiness.

BRILLIANT AT THE BASICS

Of course the hard part of the 80/20 rule is homing in on the specific 20 percent, as it's all too easy to convince ourselves that it's *all* important. Just do a quick scan of the latest wellness headlines and you'll see what I mean. Activated charcoal. Infrared saunas. Probiotic facemasks. Two-hour morning routines. No wonder you feel as if there simply aren't enough hours in the day. At first, it can be hard to separate the things that matter from those that don't, but the good news is that the 80/20 rule means that you can learn to systematically identify the things that *don't* matter, leaving you with more time and energy to focus on the things that do. By focusing on the 20 percent, you can become brilliant at the basics.

"Brilliant at the basics" is an idea attributed to late champion prize-fighter Muhammad Ali, who credited his massive success to that one primary concept. Not jumping on the latest and greatest training trend. Not a high-protein, low-carb, highly defined diet. Not doing *all the things*. Nope. Instead Ali attributed his success to getting really good at *the few basic things* that matter in boxing. Showing up at the gym. Getting in the reps. Training hard. Tuning out the nonsense. Outlasting in the process when others inevitably give up. The truth is most of us know what the basics are, but the resistance typically comes because those things are usually, well, so *basic*, so fundamentally unsexy, that they are easy to underestimate. I mean, what's the excitement in taking a walk every day or standing up and moving around every hour when there's a new fitness trend to jump on? And why just focus on adding more vegetables to every meal when you can try the newest food fad? Or why drink water when there's a new magical powder to stir into your morning beverage? We've been so conditioned to believe that the more novel, wacky, shiny, and sexy something is, the more effective it will be. But this is often far from true. Constantly adding *novel* and *new* can prevent you from stripping down to the essentials. Or, you know, actually doing the basic things at all.

The way to change, then, and the way to outlast, is to figure out which actions and habits are brilliantly basic for *you* and which align with your definition of feeling good that you determined in the Feel Good Vision exercise on page 86. Getting a handle on those specific actions and habits will allow you to better manage your time and energy and to prioritize what actually matters. No more endless to-do list or prioritization paralysis. This chapter's Make it Happen Exercise provides a blueprint for exactly how to identify your 20 percent. But before we get there, I want to tell you how to take those brilliant-at-the-basics habits and make them automatic. Allow me to tell you about the Velcro Effect.

THE VELCRO EFFECT

As I've mentioned, I used to operate under the faulty assumption that I needed more hours in the day, more discipline, and more willpower to achieve lasting results. I couldn't figure out how to maintain consistency with habits, even after I'd figured out that some things matter more than others.

As it turns out, consistency with habits has more to do with a basic behavioral principle called Cue → Behavior than with willpower or discipline. Research on habits has shown that when a behavior or action occurs in response to the same cue, and is rewarded enough times, it becomes automatic. The Cue → Habit relationship may sound complicated but it's actually quite simple. Let's break it down.

A *cue* is anything that occurs just before the behavior or action; for example, getting in your car, closing your computer, a certain time of day, or a sound, such as the doorbell ringing.

Behaviors are the things that you do; for example, taking a deep breath, heading out for a run, eating dessert, or making a cup of coffee. A *habit* is a behavior that you do so often it becomes automatic.

The more each Cue → Behavior relationship is practiced, the more your brain rewires to automate the behavior, which turns the behavior into a habit. In other words, Cue → Behavior turns into Cue → Habit, becoming so automatic that you no longer have to think about it. The powerful thing about the Cue → Habit relationship is that you can create purposeful loops in your own life so you'll need less discipline or willpower to get the same level of results.

I call the Cue → Habit relationship the Velcro Effect. Think of a cue as the hooks on Velcro, and the habit as the loops. Using the Velcro analogy, you can take any cue and stick it to a habit. Part of the magic of the Velcro Effect is that it allows you to take your 20 percent habits and then create a system to automate them. Here are a few examples of the Velcro Effect in action.

CUE: TURN ON YOUR COMPUTER
↓
HABIT: OPEN UP YOUR BROWSER AND CHECK EMAIL

CUE: FINISHING LOADING THE DISHWASHER
↓
HABIT: POUR A GLASS OF WINE

CUE: PARTNER COMES HOME FROM WORK
↓
HABIT: GO FOR A WALK

CUE: FRIDAY NIGHT
↓
HABIT: ORDER TAKEOUT

LET THIS LEAD TO THAT

You can use the Velcro Effect to automate your 20 percent habits by creating what I call Let This Lead to That rules. All you need to do is decide on a small behavior or action on which to focus. Then you'll select a cue to hook it to—either an event, time, or location—in order to make it stick. From there, you'll simply need to practice the Cue → Habit chain until it becomes automatic.

For example, having noticed a pattern of stress resulting from navigating city traffic, I created a Let This Lead to That rule to help alleviate such tension. I decided the cue would be the end of a drive, signified by taking the keys out of the ignition. Using the Velcro Effect, I chose to stick the habit of deep breathing to this cue. I defined the habit as one deep inhale and one equally long exhale, repeated three times. Here's what my Let This Lead to That rule looks like in action.

THIS: TAKE THE KEYS OUT OF THE IGNITION
↓
THAT: DEEP INHALE AND EQUALLY LONG EXHALE,
REPEATED THREE TIMES

The key here is to repeat the This → That rule as consistently as possible until it becomes automatic. So in my example, even if I'm running late to a meeting, or other people in the car might think my habit a bit strange, I continue to practice it. Keys out, inhale, exhale, repeat. That's it.

One amazing thing about using the Velcro Effect to hook these two things together is that I now get to practice breath work *and* reduce my stress, without trying to find time for an hour-long mindfulness practice. I don't have to wait for tomorrow, or for an extra hour during my morning routine. Since it's already baked in, I simply do it and move on with my day. Here are a few more examples of Let This Lead to That rules.

THIS: SIT DOWN AT THE COMPUTER
↓
THAT: DRINK A SMALL GLASS OF WATER

THIS: TURN OFF THE TELEVISION AND PREPARE FOR BED
↓
THAT: PLUG IN YOUR PHONE IN ANOTHER ROOM

THIS: FINISH THE LAST CALL OR MEETING OF THE MORNING
↓
THAT: GET UP AND TAKE A 10-MINUTE WALK

Added together, creating This → That rules will lead to a life filled with 20 percent habits, one involving less reliance on willpower or discipline alone. As you start setting your This → That rules, you'll likely begin to see many opportunities to insert them throughout your day. When you step into the shower. When you pour your first cup of coffee. When you catch the train to school.

Just note that before you go "optimizing" your entire day with This → That rules, first return to the Feel Good Mindset. Falling back into perfectionism or all-or-nothing thinking misses the point of this powerful strategy, which is not to optimize the strategy for the sake of the strategy but to use it as a means to feel good. I also recommend implementing one This → That rule at a time, as the incremental approach aligns better with mindset and method and also increases your chance of success overall. As I've said earlier, studies have shown that it's best to start by adopting one new habit at a time, working toward automation before adding additional habits.

Similarly, you'll likely find more success if you start by adding a new "good" habit, rather than trying to eliminate an old "bad" habit. So, for example, if you want to stop mindlessly scrolling on your phone, start by adding a new habit to substitute for scrolling—something such as reading a magazine, texting with family or friends, or going for a walk. Then, using the Velcro technique, create a specific cue to hook to the micro-habit. From there, practice until it becomes automatic.

WHEN YOU CAN'T PRIORITIZE WHAT MATTERS

Before moving on, I want to address something I have struggled with, and a trap I want you to avoid when it comes to the 80/20 rule. I want to talk about what to do when you feel like you can't prioritize your 20 percent. Take sleep, for example. Not to spoil the surprise but, for most people, getting a quality night's sleep is a 20 percent action that leads to results, as it contributes to feeling good in so many ways.

When you're well rested you have more energy, more patience, more focus. But for some, sleep is elusive. Whether you're struggling with an illness, little ones who aren't sleeping through the night, hormonal shifts that impact the length or quality of sleep, or a job that makes sleep difficult, if you're sleep deprived you know *exactly* how important it is. But nothing, and I mean nothing, is more frustrating than someone telling you how important sleep is when you're not getting enough of it. Because, *hello*, you are already well aware. So if this is the case for you, if you're unable to prioritize what matters for whatever reason—whether it's sleep or something else—I want you to know it's okay.

If you identify an action that you know falls into your 20 percent, but it's simply not something you can prioritize right now, the best course of action is to *let it go*. At least for the moment. Of course, if there is a way to prioritize it, then by all means, do it. But if you've tried everything, and it's still not happening, it is okay to let it go for now and instead find other ways to compensate. For example, if sleep is in your 20 percent, focus on what you can control. You might consider adding deep breathing in order to reap the immediate calming, stress-reducing effects, or try swapping a restorative yoga class for a higher-intensity workout for a while. Sleep as long as possible instead of getting up early for a morning routine. Drink more water. Clean up how you're eating. Create a core of basic actions that will allow you to feel good *and* that will work for you *right now*.

Okay, there you have it. Some actions matter more than others, and identifying those things, your own brilliant-at-the-basics habits, or your core 20 percent, will allow you to outlast by focusing your time and energy on what matters, better aligning your life with how you want to feel overall. Once you know your 20 percent, use the power of This → That rules to automate habits to support the 20 percent. Now, if you're ready to take action, I've created this chapter's Make It Happen Exercise to help you do just that.

MAKE IT HAPPEN EXERCISE: 80/20 CIRCLES

This exercise is designed to help you gain a clear understanding of how you're currently spending your time and energy and then help you identify your 20-percent habits. It's also designed to help you create This → That rules to automate your 20-percent habits.

TRACK

For two days, record as many habits and activities within your day as you can. I recommend recording at least one weekday and one weekend day. For example, every half-hour, stop and record what you're doing. You can do this in a notebook, on a piece of paper, or on your phone. If you find it difficult to remember to record, use the timer on your phone to remind you.

RANK

Referencing the tracking sheet, create a master list of all your habits and activities on the left side of a piece of paper. Next, rank each item on a scale from 1 to 3 in terms of how related that habit or activity is to your Feel Good definition that you created in the exercise on page 86, with 1 being the most related, and 3 being least related.

INNER, MIDDLE, AND OUTER CIRCLES

On a separate piece of paper, draw three concentric circles. Write the habits and behaviors that ranked a 1 in the inner circle, those that ranked a 2 in the middle circle, and those that ranked a 3 in the outer circle.

The outer circle contains the actions and habits that are *least* related to your definition of feeling good. These habits and actions are big contributors to the 80 percent, or those that aren't actually moving the needle in your life. Consider how you might reduce the amount of time or energy you're spending on them.

The middle circle contains the actions and habits that are *moderately* connected to your definition of feeling good. These habits and actions are slightly contributing to your 80 percent. Consider how you might reduce the amount of time or energy you're spending on them, or tweaking them so they better align with your definition of feeling good.

The inner circle contains the set of actions that *most* contribute to your definition of feeling good. These are your brilliant-at-the-basic actions, the 20 percent that are likely to make the biggest difference. Consider ways to prioritize these habits and actions and use This → That rules to automate them.

You might also notice that there are some key habits missing from your inner circle. If that's the case, consider how you might add habits that would better fit here.

THIS → THAT

Select one habit from your inner circle. Then identify a cue on which to hook it and create a Let This Lead to That rule. Practice until it becomes automatic, then repeat.

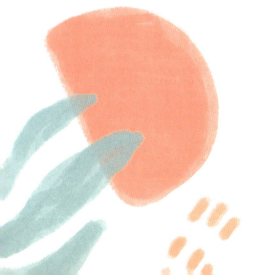

80/20 CIRCLES

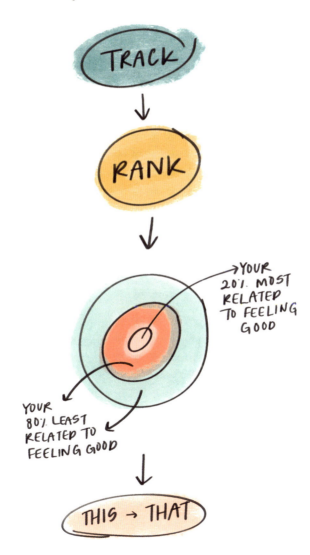

TRACK

RANK

YOUR
20% MOST
RELATED
TO FEELING
GOOD

YOUR
80% LEAST
RELATED TO
FEELING GOOD

THIS → THAT

SEVEN

Optimize to Satisfice

Have you ever struggled to make a decision, perhaps agonizing over how to make the right choice, or become trapped in analysis paralysis, overwhelmed by all the options and unable to make a choice and move forward? Making the right choice used to be a huge stumbling block for me, as I'd often get stuck in a trap of trying to make *perfect* decisions. At the time, I couldn't see that as the real problem; but looking back now, it's clear.

I fell in the perfect-decision trap a few years ago when I returned to work following maternity leave with Elle. Heading back to the office, I was determined to exclusively breastfeed, even if that meant pumping for hours on end. After a few weeks, though, pumping became a dreaded chore, and I came home depleted at the end of every day. I grappled with the decision of whether to continue, but I couldn't get past the fact that I wanted to have it all: exclusively breastfeed *and* not burn out in process. I felt a heaviness in weighing the options, and I was convinced there had to be a way to have both. I felt stuck, incapable of making the decision because I was refusing to acknowledge the pros and cons. But that's the thing. Every decision comes with a set of trade-offs. Looking back, I wish I had understood how to analyze the benefits and drawbacks and then make the *best possible* decision, rather than feeling paralyzed trying to make the *perfect* one.

In my attempt to exclusively breastfeed, I was trading time and a good amount of my sanity, yet I had zero awareness or acknowledgment of the inherent outcomes. In my mind, it seemed that there must be a perfect decision, one that would allow me to exclusively breastfeed, *and* work, *and* not spend hours pumping. Now, the point here isn't whether exclusive breastfeeding is good or bad, nor is it which option I should have chosen. The point is that there *simply is no decision without trade-offs*, no "balance" disguised as perfection.

Even if you've never been faced with this specific dilemma, my guess is you can recall a decision in your own life when you couldn't see or didn't want to recognize the give and take. Recently a friend of mine decided to relocate for work, but he quickly became frustrated by the process of moving—trying to rent his old apartment, find a new place, and handle all the hassles of packing and unpacking. The problem wasn't the move. The problem was that he'd made a decision hoping for a perfect world, one where he could move and not deal with any of the hassle. He hadn't considered and acknowledged the trade-offs, which cost him both time and frustration in the long run.

PERMISSION TO SATISFICE

So if perfect solutions don't exist, what exactly are you supposed to do? You need to *satisfice*. No, that's not a typo. While *satisficing* sounds like a made-up word, it is a very real thing. It's actually a combination of the words *satisfy* and *suffice*, coined by economist, political scientist, and cognitive psychologist Herbert Simon. Simon studied how humans make decisions, and he came to the conclusion that we can find either "optimum solutions for a simplified world, or satisfactory solutions for a more realistic world." Meaning that when the set of options are simple, you can indeed make a "perfect" choice. But when the set of options are complex, when there are countless variables, connections, and complexities, the best you can do is make a *satisfactory* choice. Not perfect. Just the best possible given the realistic alternatives.

Unfortunately, when it comes to making decisions, or choices, or the elusive quest for balance, it seems many of us still get stuck trying to find optimum solutions. But that's the problem because we don't live in a simplified world. Instead we live in one that is highly complex and connected. One where every decision contains within it many exchanges. One that requires not optimum solutions but satisfying, satisfactory solutions, which tend to counter a lot of what we often believe when it comes to decision-making. Sure, it seems as though agonizing over the perfect choice is a good idea, but research shows that maximizing, or trying to optimize the best choice, leads to all kinds of negative outcomes. For example, people who get stuck maximizing tend to be less happy and less optimistic, have lower self-esteem, and often end up regretting their decisions after making them. People who maximize also tend to get sucked into social comparison more often, and they are less confident and less satisfied with their own choices. Research also shows that people who try to maximize tend to feel an undeniable urge to do an exhaustive search of options before making a decision. For example, someone maximizing while shopping for shoes might visit every possible store, engaging in exhaustive comparison and putting a ton of time and energy into finding the perfect option. Ironically, that same person is likely to feel less satisfied with his or her choice in the long run.

On the other hand, studies show that people who satisfice make decisions based on just a few criteria that matter to them, content in finding solutions that are *good enough* given the circumstances. For example, someone satisficing might shop for shoes based on a set of criteria such as the shoes be blue, comfortable, and made to last. Once the person finds the shoe that meets these criteria, they are then satisfied and stop searching. They don't keep shopping in the hope of finding an even better option. They select what is good enough, get what they want, don't spend unnecessary time or energy making decisions, and are usually happier with their choices in the long run. Free from agonizing and analysis paralysis, satisficers simply make the best possible choice, take imperfect action, and move forward.

IT'S ALL ABOUT TRADE-OFFS

The good news here is that being a maximizer isn't a personality trait, and someone who maximizes can start to satisfice by learning a new set of skills. The first step in the process is acknowledging that there will never be a perfect choice or decision. Satisficing is simple: it's weighing the factors, acknowledging the trade-offs, and then making the best choice possible. For *you*. At that moment. Then it's about giving yourself permission to accept the trade-offs.

That "for you" part means that your best possible decisions aren't necessarily going to be the same as someone else's, because they will be made based on your values, your preferences, and how you define feeling good. Similarly, that "right now" part means that what's best now might not be best down the road. Trade-offs can change over time. As your life circumstances change, and things shift and evolve, so, too, will your best possible decisions. This takes the pressure off, allowing you to take a deep breath and let some things go. Satisficing gives you the opportunity to reframe that whole elusive concept of balance. Instead of trying to do it all, all at once, you embrace the set of trade-offs, make the best possible decision for you, and move forward. In the end, you are actually able to optimize your life simply by satisficing.

The beauty of satisficing is that you're not ignoring the impact of the choices you make, throwing caution to the wind, or making decisions without thought or consideration. With satisficing, you don't have to feel as though you're settling or accepting mediocrity. It's a strategy to embrace the context of your current life instead of fighting against it, arriving at the very best possible solution without driving yourself crazy, or setting yourself up to feel like a failure. Another benefit? Optimizing by satisficing allows you to reframe "let good enough be good enough" as the objective, rather than seeing it as settling. Because good enough *is* good enough. It's really all there is, anyway. Satisficing allows you to identify what's truly essential and then to make the best possible choice.

MAKE IT HAPPEN EXERCISE: SATISFICE CIRCLES

This exercise is designed to help you identify the trade-offs involved in any decision, which will allow you to make the best possible decision based on your values, season of life, and definition of feeling good.

SELECT A DECISION

Think about a decision you want to make. It can be something small, like figuring out how many minutes to exercise each day, or something big, like deciding if you should go back to school. Write down the decision at the top of a piece of paper.

ALL-IN AND ALL-OUT CIRCLES

Draw two large circles, slightly askew, on the paper. In the left circle, write out the case(s) for an all-in option. For example, exercising for 60 minutes every day or quitting your job to go back to school. This is your All-In circle.

Then in the right circle, write out all the extreme case(s) for the all-out option. For example, not exercising at all, or keeping your job and staying with the status quo. This is your All-Out circle.

TRADE-OFFS

Under the All-In circle, write a list of trade-offs for the case(s); that is, what will you have to give up or let go of to pursue this option. Then under the All-Out circle, write a second list of trade-offs necessary to reach this outcome. No need to overthink it; just go with whatever comes to mind first.

SATISFICE

At the bottom of the paper, draw a set of overlapping circles. This overlap is your opportunity to satisfice. Write down as many options as you can think of *in between* the two extremes.

CONSIDER THE OPTIONS

Now, looking at the circles as a whole, ask yourself the following three questions.

> Are the scenarios in the All-In circle worth the trade-offs?

This is an important question to ask, as it often reveals additional trade-offs that you may not have considered.

> Are the scenarios in the All-Out circle worth those trade-offs?

Similarly, this question is helpful as it sometimes reveals additional trade-offs that may have not been considered.

> Are there options in the Satisfice circle that represent a more satisfactory mix of trade-offs?

This step will allow you to see clearly that *all* options come with trade-offs; thus, the decision-making process becomes the act of selecting the mix that works best for you right now.

MAKE A DECISION

Once you've considered the options and trade-offs, it's time to make a decision. Again, there's no right or wrong answer; nor is there a perfect solution. You might decide to go with a scenario in the All-In circle because, after considering the trade-offs, you decide it's worth it. Similarly, you might decide to go with an All-Out option because you realize it's worth those scenarios. Sometimes satisficing means keeping things the same, at least in the short term. You might also find that there are options within the overlapping circles you may have not previously considered. Or, with a few small tweaks, you can move an All-In or All-Out option into the satisfice circles, making it far more doable and sustainable.

As you repeat this exercise with various decisions, you'll find that the process becomes easier and faster. In fact, you'll most likely find that you no longer need to draw the circles because you'll be able to weigh trade-offs in your head, make a decision, and move on without giving it a second thought. I do recommend, however, completing the exercise in full until the process becomes second nature.

satisfice circles

WHEN MAKING A
DECISION YOU
CAN GO...

ALL
IN

TRADE-OFFS

or

ALL
OUT

TRADE-OFFS

or

SATISFICE

TRADE-OFFS

THERE IS NO ONE
RIGHT DECISION

EIGHT

Decision Diet

The last part of the GOOD Method is Decision Diet. Don't worry, I'm not talking about traditional dieting here; instead, a Decision Diet is a strategy that will allow you to systematically make fewer decisions and reduce distractions, resulting in more energy and mental clarity. A Decision Diet is the solution for when you feel as though you're practically dragging yourself across the finish line, drained of willpower by the end of the day. Or those days when you manage to multitask your way through the morning, resisting the temptation to grab a triple-extra-large mocha for the morning commute, then scattering your attention across a dozen or so tasks throughout the afternoon, skipping lunch in the process because you had so many other things to do. Or days when nothing particularly out of the ordinary happens, but by 4:00 p.m. you find yourself exhausted and completely drained. As a result, even though you resisted temptations all day, you head to the vending machines to grab a bag of candy, or skip your workout in favor of an impromptu happy hour. Then, of course, you end up beating yourself up, telling yourself you just need more self-control and more willpower—to skip takeout and make dinner at home for once, to hit the gym instead of the couch, or to stop binging Netflix and pick up reading again.

Yet over and over, this much-wished-for willpower disappears around midafternoon. Every. Single. Time. The thing is, we've been conditioned to think willpower is the answer. That to create the life you want, you just need to have *more*—more discipline, more willpower, more self-control. We talk about willpower as if it's a personality trait, or a type of person; something that you either are or you're not. But guess what? Nothing could be further from the truth. Because willpower is a myth. In reality, what we typically call willpower, or self-control, is really just a form of *mental energy* that can quickly burn out in the face of too many decisions. And mental energy is a limited resource; you start the day with a certain amount and then it depletes as you spend it. And as your mental energy drains, you are more likely to follow the path of least resistance, seeking immediate gratification over sticking with your habits and goals.

FATIGUE FORMULA

Here's what's going on when it comes to willpower. As I said, it's actually just a form of mental energy that gets depleted throughout the day. There are two main culprits when it comes to mental-energy drain: decision-making and task switching. Let's talk about decision-making first.

Every time you make a small decision, it represents a tiny drain on your mental energy. This means every decision you make throughout the day compiles, which can add up to major energy depletion. It's called decision fatigue, and it's a very real thing.

Then there's task switching. Like decision-making, every time you switch your attention from one task to another—we usually call this multitasking—you drain a little more mental energy.

I call the combined energy drain of decision fatigue and task switching the Fatigue Formula.

DECISION-MAKING
+
TASK SWITCHING
=
MENTAL ENERGY DEPLETION
=
LESS WILLPOWER AND SELF-CONTROL

The Fatigue Formula represents the accumulation of decisions you make in a day, combined with the total number of times you switch attention between activities or engage in multitasking. The combination equals an overall drain of mental energy, which equates to depleted willpower and self-control. This illustrates perfectly one of the biggest problems in our modern lives, one jam-packed with decision-making opportunities and temptations to multitask. Depending on who you are and your set of life circumstances, it's quite possible you're making hundreds—if not thousands—of small decisions each day, and similarly uncountable times task switching. And if you happen to be living below the poverty threshold, the decision burden is worsened. Studies have shown that the type of decisions resulting from poverty-related concerns drains even more energy and attention.

Regardless of one's economic background, modern life poses countless decision opportunities each day. For example, studies have shown people make about 227 food decisions *per day*, most of which they are not even consciously aware. All those food decisions—what, when, and how much to eat—can really add up. Just think about some similar decisions you've probably already made today. *Should I eat in or go out? Order something? From where? What should I order? Does this dish comply with my diet? Or maybe I should cook? What should I make? Do I need to do a quick search for a recipe? Which site should I search? And which recipe should I make? Do I have these ingredients? Should I stop at the store on the way home or order online? Should I have a second helping?* And those are a few decisions you might make *just about food* within a short period of the overall day.

Likewise, think about the decisions you might make related to something as simple as exercise. The "should" internal struggle can be so real. Perhaps your inner dialogue sounds a little something like, *Should I go on a walk today? I don't really feel like it, but maybe I should because it's been a few days? What's the weather like? It's raining, so maybe I'll skip it? There's so much I need to get done. But I promised myself I'd start walking more, so maybe I should just go? If I go, what should my route be? Should I ask someone to come with me?* Notice just how many small decisions went into the quick mental debate. All that mental energy, and no actual exercise even took place.

Then add all the task switching that happens throughout the day, and it's no wonder we struggle with willpower. Task switching is one of those things that has become so ingrained that you might not even notice it's happening. But just think about the last time you sat down at your computer or opened your phone. Be honest, how many tabs or apps did you have open? Ten? Twenty? More? Now think about how many times you switched between the tasks, taking a quick look at your email, switching to check the breaking news ping, switching to your calendar tab, answering a text, switching back to a social media app, checking the news feed, and then heading back to email. Each of these switch-check-switch moments may not seem like much in the moment, but they can add up to a huge drain on your mental energy overall.

THE WILLPOWER BATTERY

Think about mental energy like the battery on your phone. Each time you use your phone, it drains a little off the battery. You've probably noticed, too, that certain apps drain a lot more battery life than others. Decision-heavy tasks and task switching are like those apps, draining far more than their fair share of your willpower battery. If you happen to be in a relationship or caring for other people, the decision and task switching load only increases. Now you are making decisions for not only yourself but also for others. *What time should I schedule her doctor's appointment? Do we have time to meet for a date this week—and if so, where should we go? Do I need to grab a birthday gift for him—and if so, what? What medication does he need today, and do I have time to pick it up on the way home from work?* With all these decisions and task switching, it's no wonder that this year for my birthday I told Andrew that all I wanted was a day not making any decisions. The depletion is so real.

DECISION TEMPLATES

By now you get the picture: Decision fatigue and task switching drain your metal energy, which means less willpower and self-control at the end of the day. But now you're probably wondering what you're supposed to do about it. You still need to respond to emails, schedule appointments, and figure out what to eat for dinner. In reality, it's impossible to stop making decisions or to eliminate task switching altogether. So that's not what I'm asking you to do. This is not an all-or-nothing situation.

Instead, I'm going to tell you how to use the Decision Diet strategy so you can navigate decision-heavy tasks and task-switching temptations with more focus and ease. A Decision Diet is about limiting your number of options *ahead of time*. It's a way to simplify and streamline, so you can structure your life to conserve mental energy, resulting in more willpower when you need it. The first step is to identify decision-heavy tasks or those with heavy task-switching temptations within your daily routines. For example, getting dressed in the morning, switching tabs or apps on your computer or phone, deciding whether to work out, or figuring out what to make for dinner. The second step is to pick one of those repeating tasks or decisions and create a Decision Template—a way to make decisions ahead of time. By paring down, you have *fewer* choices but *better* options.

One Decision Template you're probably familiar with is the capsule wardrobe. It involves examining the contents of your closet, removing anything you don't wear, and then figuring how to use the remaining pieces together, adding in additional pieces if necessary. The end result of the paring down is a curated wardrobe that includes a number of items that can be combined effortlessly for a variety of outfits, eliminating the need to spend mental energy in the process of deciding what to wear. The beauty of the capsule wardrobe as a Decision Template is that when it comes time to get dressed, most of the decisions have already been made. You've already decided that the clothes in your closet are those that you want to wear, and you've already figured out how they go together. Here are a few more examples of Decision Templates.

MEAL MAPPING

As an alternative to traditional meal planning, I create a weekly Meal Map, which serves as a Decision Template for what to eat on weeknights. Creating this template offers enough structure so that we're not constantly scrambling to figure out what's for dinner, but it still allows enough flexibility and variety to stave off boredom. For example, a Meal Map for the week might look like Monday, bowls; Tuesday, tacos; Wednesday, slow cooker; Thursday, pasta; Friday, burgers.

Developing a solid Meal Map will allow you to get creative by swapping different ingredients within the basic recipes. For example, Taco Tuesday might include chicken filling one week; beef, the following; and fish, the next. By using a Meal Map, grocery shopping is also streamlined. Write down your five to seven meals and fill in the basic ingredients under each. Just repeat weekly, modifying the ingredients slightly, while sticking to the basic framework. Fewer decisions; better results.

ESSENTIAL SIX

Another of my favorite food-related Decision Templates is what I like to call the Essential Six, or the basic building blocks of any meal, which can be mixed and matched to create a variety of options. The Essential Six include proteins, grains and bases, cooked veggies, raw veggies, sauces, and toppings and extras. Using this Decision Template, I'm able to combine the Essential Six much like one might with a capsule wardrobe.

So if it's taco night, I would select a protein (chicken), grain and base (corn tortilla), cooked veggies (pepper and onion), raw veggie (romaine lettuce), sauce (salsa), and topping (avocado). The next time I make tacos, I'd keep the same Decision Template but shuffle the Essential Six for variety. Keeping one set of variables constant reduces the decision load drastically, and it streamlines the question of what to make for dinner.

WORKOUT RULES

Creating a Decision Template for working out might look like simply deciding ahead of time when and where to work out. Because the decision's already been made, the mental debate about whether to do it is eliminated. In this case, the Decision Template might require sitting down on the weekend and looking at your calendar. What time of day is most realistic? How long is actually doable? What exactly will you do, when will you do it, and where? Making these decisions ahead might take a bit of work at first, but the beauty of a Decision Template is that it can be repeated, so you spend the energy once and reap the rewards over a long period of time.

SINGLE-TASKING BLOCKS

To alleviate the effects of task switching or multitasking, create a single-tasking Decision Template. Begin by identifying a time of day or activity when you are most tempted to switch between multiple things. Perhaps it's in the morning sitting in front of your computer, or in the afternoon scrolling apps on your phone. Next, set a specific amount of time (start small, say, 15 minutes) to focus on just one thing. This is now your single-tasking block.

Implement the block daily at the predetermined time, and reduce temptation to multitask by closing tabs and turning off notifications. Do what you can to keep distractions to a minimum. Set the timer and focus on one thing. If it's difficult, if your mind wanders, or if you feel an undeniable urge to task switch, know that's completely normal. Single-tasking is a muscle, and it takes time to build. As you get more comfortable with single-tasking, you can consider increasing your time blocks, and adding more focused blocks throughout your day.

BOUNDARIES CREATE FREEDOM

When I first introduce the concept of Decision Templates, I sometimes get pushback from people who worry that setting up boundaries and creating rules will stifle their creativity or somehow take away options. They fear that creating constraints and adding structure will feel restrictive, repressive, or boring. What I've found, though, both in the research and through teaching this method to thousands of people, is that creating a set of boundaries or rules actually *creates* freedom and options, rather than snuffing it. This is true in part because *I'm* not the one telling you which rules to create for yourself. Rather, you are creating boundaries based on your Feel Good Vision. You're in control here. This is about what works for you. Similarly, Decision Templates and the boundaries are meant to be flexible, meaning they can evolve and be tweaked over time to meet your needs. Additionally, most people find that using the Decision Diet strategy leads to so much more mental energy that they are free to spend time on what actually matters to them, versus wasting it on unnecessary decision-making and multitasking. Boundaries create freedom. It's as simple as that.

LESS WILLPOWER BY DESIGN

One more bonus is that the physical spaces and places where you spend your time have a direct influence on your ability to create and maintain healthful habits. As we wean off the idea that willpower and discipline are what we need to get results, know that your environment has a direct influence on your habits. Not willpower. Not discipline. But how your environment is set up. If things are out of sight, difficult to access, or hard to find, you're less likely to maintain the habit with which those items are associated. Conversely, when environmental barriers are removed and objects are in sight, easy to access, or simple to find, you're more likely to adopt or maintain the associated habit.

This means that you can *increase* the habits you want by removing obstructions so the habits are easier to start and maintain. Similarly, you can *decrease* habits you don't want by adding barriers, making the habit more work to maintain and therefore less likely to happen. Altering your environment to increase or decrease habits takes advantage of the fact that our brains are always looking for shortcuts, or ways to follow the path of least resistance. Even small obstacles (anything that makes you work harder) will cause you to avoid taking action. That's why something as seemingly insignificant as where you store your potato chips can actually make a big impact on your amount of snacking. It might seem obvious, as you think about it now, but the way your space is set up—what's easily available or difficult to access—makes a *huge* difference when it comes to creating and maintaining new habits.

Studies show that environment influences everything from how much water you drink to how much and when you eat. For example, just seeing a sweet treat can make you think you're hungry, even if you aren't. That explains all those fast-food commercials that suddenly appear on your screen at nine o'clock at night; right? But, if you create an environment full of healthful food, your brain and body will actually learn to crave that food over time. Even something as simple as the size of your bowl or plate can make a difference, research shows. In one study, people were given a small (8-ounce) or large (12-ounce) bowl and invited to serve themselves as much ice cream as they wanted. The people who had the large bowl served themselves and ate a lot more ice cream than people with the small bowl. It didn't matter if the people were on a diet, or had better willpower or better motivation. The *only* factor that differentiated the two groups was the size of the bowl.

CLEAR FOR MORE

To start or maintain a habit, think about ways to make it easier. Clear the way to make it the most obvious option. Make it simple. Do it more. For example:

> If you want to eat more vegetables, place them on the center shelf of your refrigerator rather than the back of the crisper drawer.
>
> If you want to go to the gym more often, prepack a gym bag and put it next to your car keys the night before, place a pair of comfortable walking shoes and socks by the front door, or store a spare set of workout clothes in the back of your car or commute bag.

If you want to be more consistent with stretching, put a yoga mat in front of your television.

If you want to drink more water, fill a clear pitcher with water at the beginning of the day, put a big glass and the pitcher on your desk or countertop, and make sure the pitcher is empty by the end of the day.

OUT OF SIGHT FOR LESS

To quit or reduce an undesirable habit, think about ways to make it harder to happen. Intentionally create barriers, add more steps, make it harder to physically access, or remove it from view. For example:

If you want to reduce the amount of time on your phone, charge it in a different room or, better yet, plug it in inside a cabinet.

If you want to decrease a fast-food habit, change your route home, avoiding your biggest temptations.

WHEN DECISIONS ARE YOUR JOB

A quick note here, before we move on, to address a frequently asked question about the Decision Diet strategy: What if decision-making and task switching are integral to your job? If this is your situation, my suggestion is twofold.

First, I recommend using the Decision Diet *outside* of work to start. Focus on your home environment, your commute, and the spaces and places you spend time when you're not at work. Similarly, start with Decision Templates for the early morning, evening, and weekends. Second, consider if there are small opportunities for Decision Templates at work. Even a 15-minute single-tasking block can go a long way.

MAKE IT HAPPEN EXERCISE: DECISION DIET

Using Decision Templates and environmental design together adds up to a Decision Diet, which will allow you to simplify, streamline, and conserve mental energy so you don't need to rely on willpower and discipline to develop and maintain healthful habits. Start small, focus in, tweak, experiment, and add as you go.

IDENTIFY A PROBLEM AREA

Start by mentally walking through your daily and weekly routines. Then, on a piece of paper, brainstorm a list of possible decision-heavy or multitasking "problem areas," or places where you find making decisions or multitasking time-consuming, difficult, or overwhelming. For example, deciding what to wear in the morning, when to work out, what to make for dinner, or when to answer emails.

CREATE A DECISION TEMPLATE

Pick one problem area, such as what to make for dinner, and then write out a Decision Template, or set of rules, to pre-make some of the required decisions. For example, create a Meal Map for weekday dinners. See pages 124 to 127 for more Decision Template examples.

DESIGN

Consider ways to use environmental design to make your Decision Template habits easier and more accessible. Remember Clear for More, and Out of Sight for Less.

IMPLEMENT

Implement your new Decision Template by trying it out. You may find it works well, or you may find that the rules you came up don't quite work yet. If you're struggling to adhere to the template, or if it seems overly complicated, adjust and simplify. Know that it might take some experimentation to get it right, so continue to tweak and adjust until it feels intuitive. Then repeat the process with other problem areas.

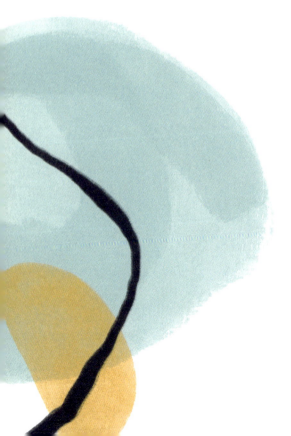

decision diet

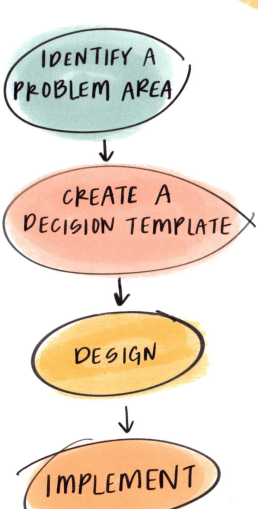

IDENTIFY A PROBLEM AREA

CREATE A DECISION TEMPLATE

DESIGN

IMPLEMENT

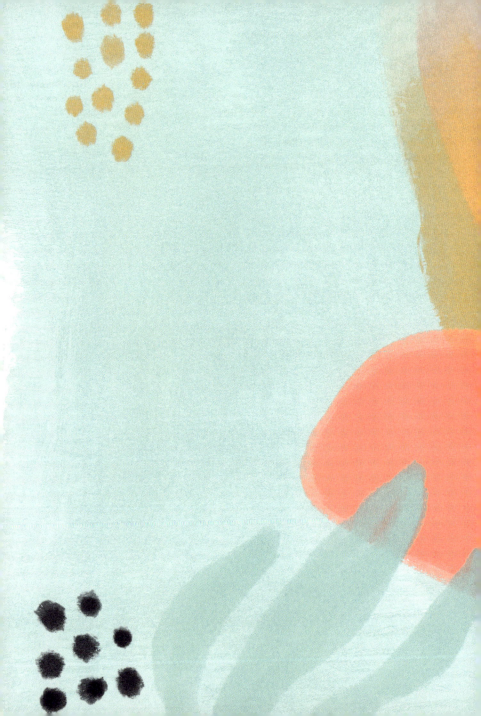

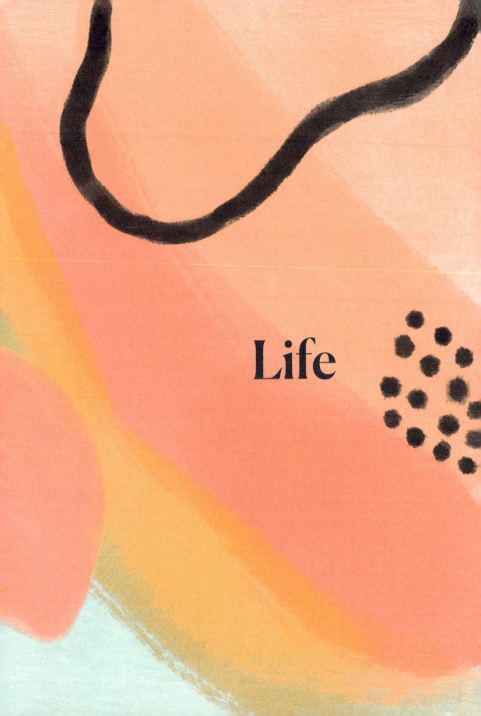

Life

NINE

The Feel Good Life

When Andrew and I got married almost two decades ago, we decided to write our own vows. Stuck on what to say, I conferred with my dad, asking him if I could borrow from the vows he had written for my mom more than forty years earlier. From those forty-year-old wedding vows I took the following line: "I have only one life, and it is only so long, and I choose to spend it with you." Now I'd like to share part of those vows with you too.

> You have only one life.
>
> It is only so long.
>
> I hope you'll spend it feeling good.

I hope you'll choose to spend it stepping away from striving. I hope you'll spend it in pursuit of the freedom and power that come from learning to treat yourself with kindness and compassion, to create days filled with gratitude, and to embrace the shades of gray. I hope you'll use the strategies and exercises in this book to work within the context of your life, instead of fighting against it.

I hope you'll own who you are, without feeling as though your life has to look like someone else's, and give up the idea that you need to be more disciplined and find more willpower. I hope you'll find more calm, more clarity, and also more joy.

I hope you'll use the tools in this book to streamline, simplify, and find more ease. To better handle the daily ups and downs, to find peace within your choices, and to know that your life isn't going to look like anyone else's—because that's what makes it beautiful, because that's what makes it yours. To define the true meaning of health, happiness, and feeling good for yourself, and to experience the incredible power of small shifts.

And I hope you'll start right now—knowing that there's no need to wait for January, or Monday, or next month. You now know you don't have to wait for perfect. Starting now; making tiny, incremental steps; and finding a radical commitment and consistency will allow you to move forward sustainably, on your time, at your pace. I hope you'll decide that it's time to show up, to do the work, to know that you are completely capable. You and I may never meet in real life, but I know these following things for sure.

You deserve this life.

You deserve to enjoy the process, to find the ease, to allow for space.

You deserve to reframe what success looks like. For you. Right now.

You deserve to feel good.

Not only do you deserve it, but so do the people and community around you. My hope is that you'll use the Feel Good Effect in your own life and allow the work to ripple outward, spreading and positively impacting other areas of work, family, relationships, and community. I believe that one of the greatest gifts I have given Elle is to live the Feel Good Effect myself; teaching her by example that there is an alternative to striving. Showing her that perfectionism, all-or-nothing thinking, and comparison need not be the default mode of operation in her own life. I'm teaching her that she can work smarter, creating a life with joy, ease, purpose, and contribution based on what works for her.

I believe that living the Feel Good Effect has made me a better partner and friend, and allowed me to contribute in ways I never thought possible. I believe the same for you. Take what you've learned in these pages and share it with the people in your life who can benefit from this shift.

Be the change.

Be the ripple.

Start right here, right now, right where you are.

A few final words of encouragement. The Feel Good Effect, at its core, is a powerful system of small shifts, a consistent process and practice. This book is here for you as a lifelong resource for support and guidance. Come back to it whenever you need a reset, some direction, or a few words of inspiration.

And don't feel as if you have to go it alone. Change often comes as part of community, so don't be afraid to create a structure of support. Make a Feel Good Effect book club. Use the resources available at realfoodwholelife.com/fgebook. Start right now by committing to the Feel Good Effect Challenge on page 141. Start with the small shifts; then watch how everything changes.

Here's to feeling good.

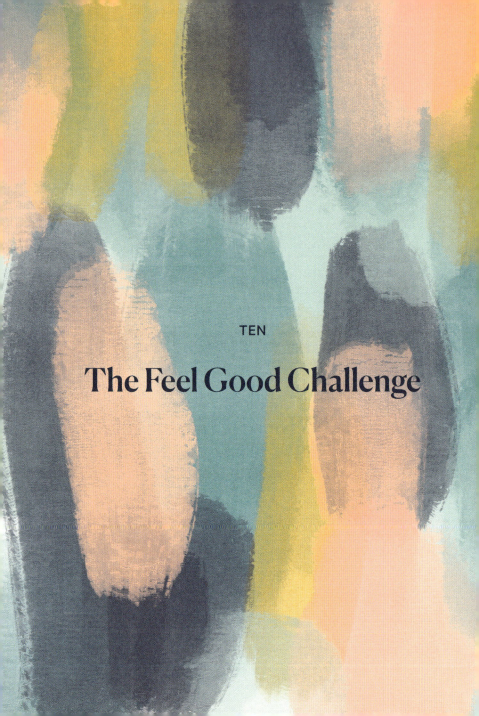

TEN

The Feel Good Challenge

Welcome to the Feel Good Challenge! I want to make your path to living the Feel Good Effect as easy as possible, so I've designed this challenge to help you take the momentum you've built and to start taking daily action. Like the entire Feel Good Effect approach, this challenge is not about perfection, all-or-nothing, or comparison. Instead, it's about taking imperfect action, making it work in your life, and doing it more days than not.

For a downloadable Feel Good Challenge workbook, visit realfood wholelife.com/fgebook.

THE CHALLENGE

Since having a game plan can be helpful when adopting a new approach, this challenge is designed to give you the exact steps to get started. If you want an autopilot version, this is it. Of course, there's always room for flexibility, so if something about the plan doesn't work, feel free to customize. Either way, to get big results, start with small steps. Change comes through commitment and consistency, and this challenge is your first move.

Before starting the Feel Good Challenge, set aside an hour and a half (all at once, or divided) to complete Steps 1 to 5.

Step 1. Take the Feel Good Effect Archetype Quiz
The quiz on page 144 typically takes 5 to 10 minutes to complete and will determine your Feel Good Effect Archetype. Keep in mind there are no right or wrong answers, so simply choose the answer that is most true for you right now.

Step 2. Find Your Feel Good Effect Archetype
After you've completed the quiz, use the Quiz Scoring Guide to determine your archetype: Dynamo, Seeker, or Cultivator. If your results are split evenly, read through the descriptions and then select the one that best describes you.

Step 3. Vision

Complete the Feel Good Vision exercise on page 86. This typically takes 15 to 30 minutes.

Step 4. Goal Flip

Once you've completed the Vision exercise, use the Goal Flip exercise on page 98 to reverse engineer a result and set Mini-Milestones and Big Wins for the next 30 days. This exercise typically takes 15 to 30 minutes.

Step 5. Mindset Practice

Use your Feel Good Effect Archetype to determine your Mindset Practice for the next 30 days.

Dynamo: 5-Minute Morning (see page 61)
Seeker: Third Way (see page 69)
Cultivator: Three Grateful Things (see page 74)

Step 6. Commitment and Consistency

Commit to consistency by setting aside 10 minutes each morning for 30 days for your Mindset Practice. If this timeframe or time of day doesn't work, customize as needed.

Step 7. Thirty Days to Feel Good

For the next month, focus on your Feel Good Effect by using your Mindset Practice and Goal Flipping. Write down your thoughts to document your progress.

BUILD IN ACCOUNTABILITY

Team up with a friend, family member, or coworker to do the challenge together, increasing your accountability.

BEYOND THE THIRTY DAYS

Once you've completed the challenge, set aside 20 to 30 minutes to reflect on your process and progress for the month. Repeat the challenge with the same Mindset Practice, or add a new practice. Keep going with your Goal Flip documentation, or select a different result as needed. Maintain your commitment to a consistent practice, adding and tweaking as you go.

THE FEEL GOOD EFFECT ARCHETYPE QUIZ

1 How would your best friend describe your approach to life?

    a. "Such an amazing friend, though sometimes gets defeated when not doing as well as other people."

    b. "So good at so many things, but sometimes a little discouraged when something isn't exactly right from the start."

    c. "Always up for something new, often before mastering a previous attempt . . . maybe needs a little help finding a middle ground and sticking with it."

2 What's one of the best things about being you?

    a. I really care about other people and value their opinions.

    b. I'm usually pretty good at everything I do.

    c. I'm usually up for trying something new and when I do, I go all-in.

3 You set a new workout goal but then get sick and miss a week of training. Feeling a bit discouraged, you tell yourself:

    a. Well that obviously didn't work. Maybe it's a sign I need to try something different.

    b. I can figure out everything else, so why can't I figure this out?

    c. Everybody else seems to be able to stick to their goals; why can't I?

4 What's exhausting about being you?

    a. Sometimes I set unrealistic goals for myself, and I can be a bit of an overthinker, which can stand in the way of taking action.

    b. I love committing to go all-in, but sometimes I burn myself out or fall off the wagon.

    c. I sometimes get distracted by what everyone else is doing; and to be honest, that can make me feel like giving up.

5 You finally save enough money to buy a new car. What are your thoughts?

    a. I'm already set on what I want. But if I can't find exactly what I'm looking for, I keep looking, even if that means never actually making the purchase.

    b. I've read all the customer reviews, plus I've considered what my friends are driving. I'm pretty sure if it works for them, it will work for me.

    c. I've done *all the research*, pored over all the websites, and found as much info as possible on everything from safety and fuel efficiency to functionality and price . . . but when it comes to actually buying a car, it's possible I'll feel there still might be a better choice.

QUIZ SCORING GUIDE

1.	a. Cultivator		3.	a. Seeker		5.	a. Seeker
	b. Dynamo			b. Dynamo			b. Dynamo
	c. Seeker			c. Cultivator			c. Cultivator
2.	a. Cultivator		4.	a. Dynamo			
	b. Dynamo			b. Seeker			
	c. Seeker			c. Cultivator			

THE FEEL GOOD EFFECT ARCHETYPES

You've discovered your Feel Good Effect Archetype; now explore your primary Striving Mindset block.

DYNAMO

You're most likely a highly motivated achiever who thrives on ticking items off the to-do list and being in charge. You know how to get things done, and when you do something, you know how to do it right—whether it's getting a scratch-made dinner on the table, taking a company public, or never missing a workout. Any project is completely safe in your hands, which is why you've got so many projects going on. You've got seriously high standards, so if you can't do it 100 percent right, why do it at all? You might put a lot of pressure on yourself to meet those standards; and when that doesn't happen, you sometimes beat yourself up. And with all you have going on, working out or eating healthfully can turn into just another item on the to-do list. This can be exhausting, especially when you're busy taking care of everything and everyone else.

SEEKER

As a Seeker you love a good trend, but to you they're not trends. A new routine, workout, or way of eating reenergizes your life—and you throw yourself into it with wild abandon. Running? Sure . . . in spurts. But you've never figured out a way to make it stick. The ketogenic diet? You'll go keto for a few months—and then forget about it. I mean, who wants to live without carbs, anyway? Crossfit was the perfect solution—before the responsibilities started piling up. Now getting to the gym seems impossible. And you *may* just have fitness equipment (plus a few memberships) gathering dust. You're an open person—and you have no fear when it comes to trying new things. But sometimes newness has a way of capturing your attention, and before you know it you're off to master the Next Best Thing. What about finding a middle ground and staying with it long term without burning yourself out? That might be just what you need right now.

CULTIVATOR

You're a super-conscientious person who cares a lot about others. Sometimes you can care so much, though, that you might struggle with feeling too much like a people pleaser. Then there's that habit of looking outside yourself for answers, which can invite comparison and FOMO (fear of missing out). All that searching can leave you feeling ungrounded, without a core structure for your life. You may even compare yourself to a different version of you from the past, which halts forward progress and can leave you feeling miserable. But what worked for you ten (or even two) years ago might not work now. Sit with that for a sec. Finding what resonates for you *right now*—not the old you, or your best friend, or the peeps out there on social media—is going to be a big deal. The thing is, we all have inner wisdom; you just sometimes doubt yours. But think about it. Our bodies are often the first in line to tell us what we need. When you tune in and take a good, hard look, chances are you already know what needs to go, what can stay, and what actually brings you joy.

Acknowledgments

The thing about rewiring your brain toward gratitude is that you begin to see gratitude everywhere. These acknowledgments are really just an extension of my own personal gratitude practice.

Gratitude to the Real Food Whole Life and Feel Good Effect podcast community. This book would not have possible without you. Thank you for reading and listening; thank you to each of you who experienced the Feel Good Effect in your own life and then worked to spread the mission and message outward. Words cannot express my humble appreciation.

To my agent, Laura Lee Mattingly, for believing in this mission and message, for your thoughtful feedback throughout, and for your commitment to representing authors with perspectives that challenge the status quo.

To my editor, Kelly Snowden, for championing this project from the beginning, for your guidance throughout the process, and for your insightful—sometimes hilarious—comments and feedback.

To my copy editor Janet Silver Ghent for exquisite attention to detail, Annie Marino for a thoughtful beautiful design, Doug Ogan for the editorial work, and to the entire team at Ten Speed Press.

To Briana Summers, for bringing the Feel Good Effect to life through your gorgeous illustrations, patterns, and washes.

To my dad, David, for giving me a brain that thinks in frameworks and models—one that never seems to turn off (thanks a lot for that last part). Gratitude for reminding me that I'm capable of great things, for your endeavors on student success, and for all the ways your work has influenced mine. Also, for your homemade margaritas and serving as my unofficial, unpaid CTO.

To my mom, Judy, for your unwavering and constant encouragement throughout, for your central role as anchor parent, for raising your daughters to be strong and powerful and kind and compassionate, and for all the ways you sacrificed to make opportunity possible for us. Also, for being my very first email subscriber and the absolute best grandma, ever.

To my, sisters, Laurel and Genevieve, and the next generation of Conley women; Ayla, Lily, and Evelyn.

Gratitude to the many phenomenal public teachers and educators who have helped shape who I am, especially those from Oregon's South Eugene High School and International High School and the Special Education Department at Central Washington University. Also to public libraries for providing access to books, especially during times in my own life when buying new books wasn't an option.

To all my fierce founder friends and virtual colleagues who, while working to change the world, manage to support me through the ups and downs of business building and authorship, including Taesha Butler, Kait Hurley, Ali Edwards, Ashley Neese, and Sonja Overhiser.

To the incredibly thoughtful and supportive women of my book club—Leah, Amy, Sharon, Diedra, Jennifer, Lisa, Heather, Erin, Jill, and Amy—and my most beautiful friendships, including Erin Vranas, Kelli Greenwald, and Julianna Gassman Hayes.

Gratitude to my city, Portland, Oregon, for endless inspiration and for providing a backdrop for a different kind of wellness, including Powell's Books, Forest Park, Grand Central Bakery (gratitude for endless coffee refills), and YoYo Yogi; as well as the fitness and wellness community, especially the studios and instructors who are changing the fitness conversation and creating space for real health and happiness.

To Elle, my smart, fierce, strong-willed, kind, loving girl—you are my greatest teacher. You taught me courage before you were ever born and then taught me to slow down and find self-compassion after. Thank you for reminding me to let go of the daily weight of endless to-do lists in favor of presence, in favor of being, in favor of now. It's you, my Elle, who teaches me that time is our most precious resource, that gentle is the only option, and that since this is the only moment we've got, we ought to spend it doing the things that really matter.

Finally, to Andrew. You are the reason this is possible. This book. This work. This life. All of it. Thank you for always saying "Yes." When I say, "Here's this crazy idea I have," you say "Yes." And when I say, "Will you please collaborate with me on this research so I can write a book?" you say "Yes." And when I say, "I am having a crisis of confidence and I don't believe in myself right now, can you please believe in me on my behalf?" you say "Yes." And for the million other "yeses" you have said and will continue to say. Thank you for always standing beside me, and also behind me, together, equal; for your willingness to serve behind-the-scenes. Thank you for choosing to spend this life with me. I am forever grateful.

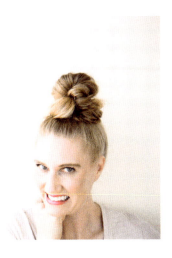

About the Author

Robyn Conley Downs is the founder of mission-driven media-and-education brand Real Food Whole Life, and creator of the Feel Good Effect Mindset & Method. She holds a master's degree in education with an emphasis in behavior change, has four years of public policy and health change at the doctoral level, and her work taps into cutting-edge science around mindset, strategies and habits, and how to create health, happiness, and sustainable wellness. She combines her professional research background with work as a certified yoga teacher—specializing in mindfulness and self-compassion—to share science-based, life-tested, radically simple solutions to help people feel good. When not writing or speaking, Robyn can be found behind the mic of the Feel Good Effect podcast, in the kitchen creating simple real-food recipes, hiking, reading, or practicing yoga in and around her home in Portland, Oregon, along with her husband, Andrew, and their daughter, Elle.

Index